I0482742

Health and Safety Awareness

Future Performance Training Academy

Dr. M Schutte (Ph.D, Msc.B)

Version 1.1

Learner Guide

COPYRIGHT

Developed by Future Performance Training Academy

Copyright Future Performance Training (Pty) Ltd. All rights reserved

No part of this Publication may reproduced, stored in retrieval system, or transmitted, in any form or by any means, electronic, mechanical, photocopying, recording or otherwise, without the prior permission of the copyright owner.

Although every attempt has been made to ensure that the management guidelines are safe and correct, the developer, publishers, and sponsors of the manual cannot accept any responsibility for errors arising from the use of this manual for any purpose.

LIMITATION OF LIABILITY

Every effort has been made to ensure complete and accurate information concerning the material presented in this course. Neither Future Performance Training Academy nor its agents can be held legally responsible for any mistakes in printing or for faulty instructions contained within this course. The publisher appreciates receiving notice of any errors or misprints.

Information in this manual is subject to change without notice. Companies, names and data used in examples herein are fictitious unless otherwise noted.

Published by Future Performance Training (Pty) Ltd

Printed by Amazon

www.amazon.com

ISBN-13: 978-1499685640
ISBN-10: 1499685645

Published 26-05-2014

This book is available to use as part of your training, teaching or learning experience and is available for sale by:

Future Performance Training (Pty) Ltd

www.futureperformance.co.za

Email: admin@futureperformance.co.za

Contact: 0393120395 / or at Amazon at www.amazon.com

Contents

Course Overview

This course introduces you to the concept of health and safety in an overall context necessary at home and work. You will learn about HIV/Aids, Health and Safety as well as how to save a life.

This course is accredited and you will be able to become a health and safety officer or a first aider once you have completed this course.

Course Outcomes

After you have completed this course you will be able to:

1. Become aware of HIV/Aids and its impact on society
2. Apply Health and Safety in your environment
3. Perform basic life support and first aid procedures

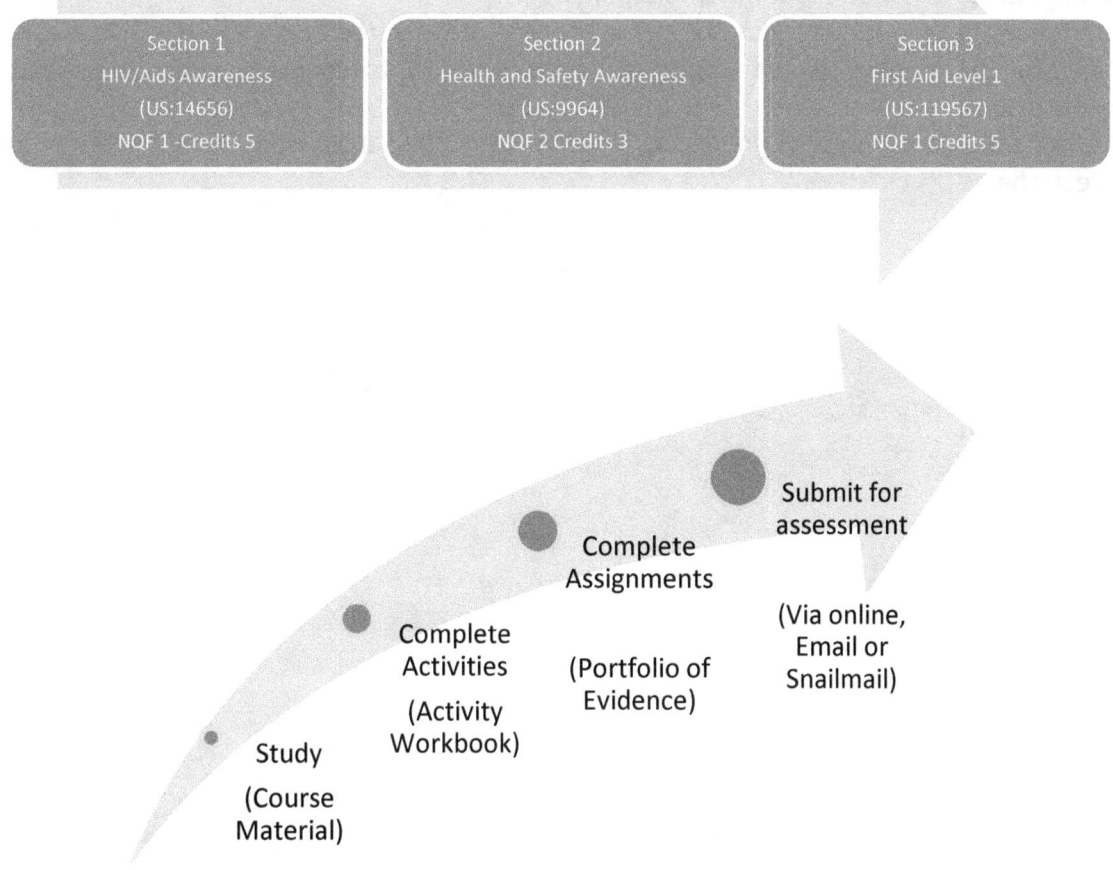

Section 1	Section 2	Section 3
HIV/Aids Awareness	Health and Safety Awareness	First Aid Level 1
(US:14656)	(US:9964)	(US:119567)
NQF 1 -Credits 5	NQF 2 Credits 3	NQF 1 Credits 5

Study
(Course Material)

Complete Activities
(Activity Workbook)

Complete Assignments
(Portfolio of Evidence)

Submit for assessment
(Via online, Email or Snailmail)

SECTION 1 - HIV/AIDS AWARENESS

Course Overview

Since Aids was first recognized in 1981, it has led to the deaths of more than 25 million people, making it one of the most destructive diseases in recorded history. This course creates an awareness of HIV/Aids amongst people and how to prevent it. This course is essential for the survival of the human race.

Course Outcomes

After you have completed this section you will be able to:

- Demonstrate an understanding of sexuality
- Demonstrate an understanding of sexually transmitted infections including HIV/AIDS
- Describe the means to cope and deal with sexually transmitted infections including HIV/AIDS
- Describe human rights of individuals living with HIV/AIDS and sexually transmitted infections

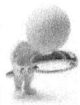

Go through the following table, this is an indication of what you will be expected to know and demonstrate an understanding in. Once you have completed this course return to this section and assess whether you grasp each specific outcome.

Specific Outcome	Assessment Criteria	Yes	No
1. Demonstrate an understanding of sexuality.	• I am able to identify the different sexual orientations and preferences with reference to community values and perceptions and attitudes towards these. • I am able to identify the rights and responsibilities in protecting sexuality with reference to the South African Constitution.		
2. Demonstrate an understanding of the nature, transmission and prevention of sexually transmitted infections including HIV/AIDS.	• I am able to explain the terms "STIs", "STDs", "HIV", "AIDS". • I am able to explain the nature and symptoms of sexually transmitted infections including HIV/AIDS according to possible ways of infection. • I am able to explain the risk taking behaviours, and preventive methods and practices regarding the transmission routes of sexually transmitted infections, including HIV/AIDS. • I am able to describe the role of sexually transmitted infections in the transmission of HIV, and an indication is given of how untreated STIs greatly increase the risk of transmission. • I am able to list the ways in which mother to child transmission can occur and the implications of pregnant women having unprotected sex are indicated for both the mother and the unborn child. • I am able to demonstrate interpersonal skills that help to reduce the risk of sexually transmitted infections, including HIV infection, in terms of assertive communication, negotiation and decision-making. • I am able to explain the importance of pre and post-test counselling and the implications of HIV testing for an individual are discussed in terms of making a personal decision to take an AIDS test. • I am able to discuss the importance of lifestyle changes to boost the immune system, with reference to diet and stress management.		
3. Describe means to cope and deal with sexually transmitted infections including HIV/AIDS.	• I am able to explain living with HIV/AIDS and other sexually transmitted with reference to the impact on the infected and the affected individuals within the context of self, family, community, workplace and society. • I am able to describe support towards people living with HIV/AIDS and sexually transmitted infections to determine the social support systems for the infected and the affected. • I am able to list available treatments for people living with HIV/AIDS and sexually transmitted infections referring to current and available medical, herbal treatments and other legal and safe practices.		

	• I am able to discuss the benefits of an organisation's HIV/AIDS policy with reference to the reduction of prejudice and discrimination against infected persons, and the removal of stigma from the disease.		
Describe human rights of individuals living with HIV/AIDS and other sexually transmitted infections.	• I am able to identify the rights and responsibilities of the infected and affected according to the Constitution and Acts that protect these rights. • I am able to examine the violation of human rights of the infected and the affected according to beliefs and attitudes towards sexually transmitted infections in the workplace and society.		

Affected employee: an employee who is affected in any way by HIV/AIDS e.g. if they have a partner or a family member who is HIV positive.

AIDS: AIDS is the acronym for "acquired immune deficiency syndrome". AIDS is the clinical definition given to the onset of certain life-threatening infections in persons whose immune systems have ceased to function properly as a result of infection with HIV.

Epidemiological: The study of disease patterns, causes, distribution and mechanisms of control in society.

HIV: HIV is the acronym for "human immune deficiency virus". HIV is a virus which attacks and may ultimately destroy the body's natural immune system.

HIV testing: taking a medical test to determine a person's HIV status. This may include written or verbal questions inquiring about previous HIV tests; questions related to the assessment of 'risk behavior' (for example questions regarding sexual practices, the number of sexual partners or sexual orientation); and any other indirect methods designed to ascertain an employee's or job applicant's HIV status.

HIV positive: having tested positive for HIV infection.

Infected employee: an employee who has tested positive for HIV or who has been diagnosed as having HIV/AIDS.

Informed consent: a process of obtaining consent from a patient which ensures that the person fully understands the nature and implications of the test before giving his or her agreement to it.

Policy: a document setting out an organisation's position on a particular issue.

Pre and post-test counseling: a process of counseling which facilitates an understanding of the nature and purpose of the HIV test. It examines what advantages and disadvantages the test holds for the person and the influence the result, positive or negative, will have on them.

Reasonable Accommodation: means any modification or adjustment to a job or to the workplace that is reasonably practicable and will enable a person living with HIV or AIDS to have access to or participate or advance in employment.

STDs: acronym for "sexually transmitted diseases". These are infections passed from one person to another during sexual intercourse, including syphilis, gonorrhea and HIV.

Surveillance Testing: This is anonymous, unlinked testing which is done in order to determine the incidence and prevalence of disease within a particular community or group to provide information to control, prevent and manage the disease.

AIDS

AIDS stands for: Acquired - not inherited; Immuno - relating to the body's immune system which provides protection from disease-causing germs; Deficiency - lack of immune response to germs; Syndrome - a number of signs and symptoms indicating a particular disease or condition. This is caused by a germ or virus called HIV. HIV can only live in blood, sperm and other bodily fluids.

HIV

Human Immunodeficiency Virus attacks the immune system and gradually destroys it. The

body cannot defend itself against infections and this results in the condition known as AIDS. The HIV germ is passed on from one person to another person through sex, blood or exchange of bodily fluids. It then begins to attack the body from the inside.

STD – Sexual Transmitted Disease

Refers to infections that are causing symptoms is an illness that is transmitted between humans by means of human sexual behaviour.

STI – Sexual Transmitted Infection

Refers to an infection with any germ that can cause an STD.

What is HIV?

In 1985, scientists discovered the human immunodeficiency virus (HIV). HIV is a virus that is transmitted from one person to another through the exchange of body fluids such as:

- blood
- semen
- breast milk
- vaginal secretions

As well as through direct contact with the Mucous Membrane such as:

- mouth
- nose
- eyes

- penis
- anus
- vagina

Sexual (anal, oral and vaginal) contact is the most common way to spread HIV AIDS, but it can also be transmitted by:

- sharing needles when injecting drugs
- blood transfusions
- pregnancy
- during childbirth
- breastfeeding

As HIV AIDS reproduces, it damages the body's immune system and the body becomes susceptible to illness and infection. Acquiring one of these infections means a person is diagnosed with AIDS.

A person can be infected for years without having AIDS. Having HIV infection does not mean you have AIDS. HIV and AIDS are not the same thing.

HIV cannot be transmitted through casual contact. Personal contact in the workplace, at home or at school is casual.

You cannot get HIV by any of the following activities:

- patting someone on the back
- sharing equipment
- sharing restrooms
- shaking hands
- hugging
- coughing
- sneezing
- using the same drinking fountain
- using the same telephone
- eating together

There is no risk of transmission from:

- saliva, sweat, tears, urine,
- respiratory droplets, handshaking, swimming-pool water, communal bath
- water, toilets, food or drinking water

Research shows that family members of people with HIV/AIDS have not been infected with the virus through normal household contact. Even people who have bathed or slept in the same bed with HIV/AIDS patients have not become infected.

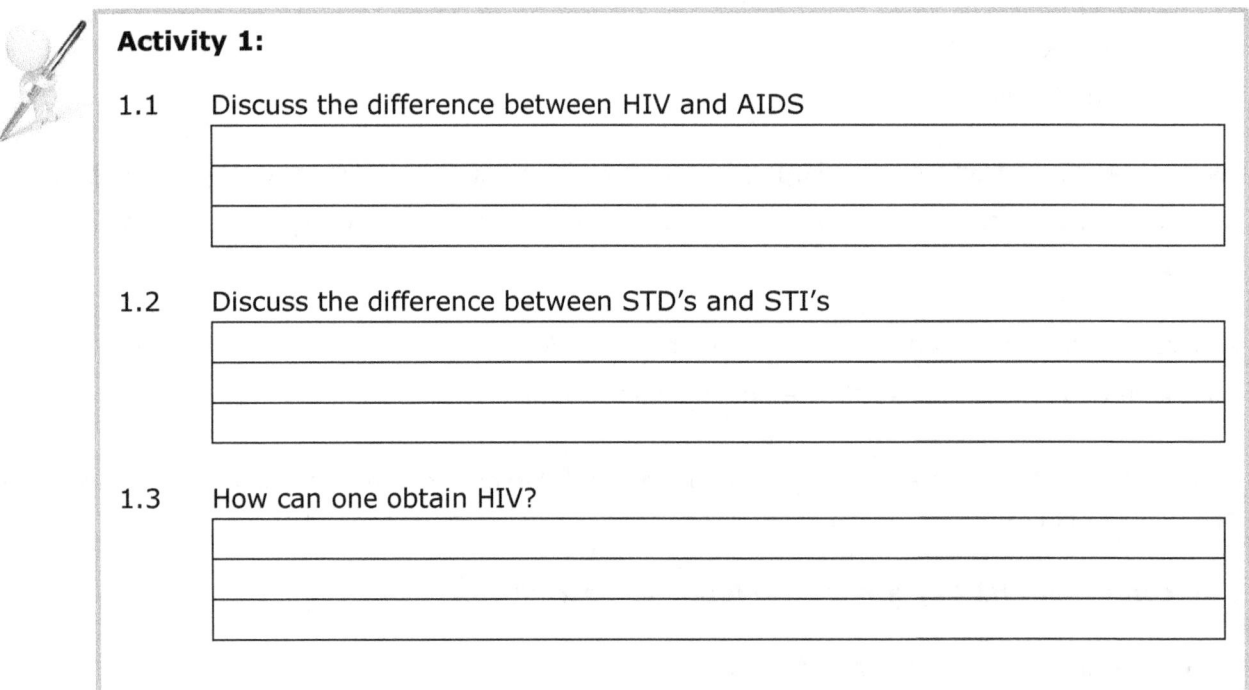

Activity 1:

1.1   Discuss the difference between HIV and AIDS

1.2   Discuss the difference between STD's and STI's

1.3   How can one obtain HIV?

The Importance of Understanding what HIV/AIDS is?

By understanding the HIV virus, the chance of living a healthier, longer life increases. In the beginning of the epidemic, an AIDS diagnosis signalled death would soon follow. But today, thanks to the development of HIV medications, people are no longer dying from AIDS they are living with the HIV virus. To live a productive, healthy life with HIV, one must learn as much as possible about the disease.

South Africa has the largest population of HIV patients in the world. It is estimated that almost 25% of South Africa's population is infected by the HIV virus.

HIV/AIDS prevalence among sexually active South Africans by province are:

- KwaZulu-Natal: 25.8%
- Mpumalanga: 23.1%
- Free State: 18.5%
- North West: 17.7%
- Gauteng: 15.2%
- Eastern Cape: 15.2%
- Limpopo: 13.7%
- Northern Cape: 9.2%
- Western Cape: 5.3%

How Does the HIV Virus Multiply?

Once inside the body the virus attacks specialized immune system cells known as CD4 cells. CD4 cells are a type of white blood cell that fights infections. CD4 cells move throughout the body, helping to identify and destroy germs such as bacteria and viruses. The HIV virus attaches to these cells and infects them by injecting HIV proteins (DNA and RNA) into the cell. The new HIV virus then infects other CD4 cells as the cycle repeats itself.

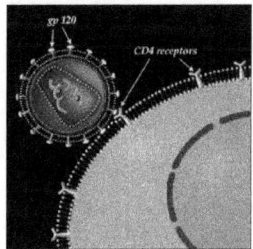 This figure illustrates how the HIV Virus attacks the immune system cells

HIV targets CD4 cells by:

- Binding to the surface of CD4 cells
- Entering CD4 cells and becoming a part of them. As CD4 cells multiply to fight infection, they also make more copies of HIV
- Continuing to replicate, leading to a gradual decline of CD4 cells

How Does the HIV Virus Harm the Body?

As the HIV virus reproduces, the CD4 cells are damaged, becoming unable to fight infections. As this process continues, the body's immune system weakens and the infected person becomes susceptible to a score of different infections, all capable of making the person sick and in extreme cases can lead to death.

What Can Be Done to Stop the HIV Virus?

While there is no cure for HIV, medications are now available that diminish the virus's ability to reproduce. This in turn helps the immune system stay healthy and able to fight infection. Keep in mind that these medications can't rid the body entirely of HIV and people can still infect others while on medications.

The reason why HIV is still spreading is because:

- People are uneducated about HIV/AIDS and how it is transmitted
- People are afraid to speak up when they think they might have it
- People still have unprotected sex
- People are unfaithful to each other
- Poverty
- Not being able to get help (clinic or health centre)
- Unequal relationships between men and woman

Unequal relationships between men and woman

In most communities, women are expected to agree to their male partners' demands and decisions. It is hard for women in these situations to say what they want or do not want.

For example, a woman who knows that her partner has other girlfriends may still not be able to ask him to use a condom. Or a woman may be afraid that her partner will abuse her if she talks about safe sex.

Poverty

Although poverty may make people more vulnerable to HIV and AIDS, poverty does not cause the disease. Poverty means that people often have to leave home to find work in other places. When people move around, they look for new friends and sometimes seek comforting.

If people worked in the same place all the time, they would find it easier to keep to one partner. This would mean that HIV and AIDs would not be spread so fast.

Poor women often struggle to find work. Sometimes they have to exchange sex for food or money. These women may not be able to insist that their clients wear condoms. When these things happen, HIV and AIDS can are spread quickly.

Poor access to health services

Some people have to travel long distances to get to the clinic. Or they may not be able to afford to go to the clinic, and so they may leave a sexually transmitted infection untreated. Having an untreated STI can make it easier for a person to get HIV.

In addition, staff at busy and overcrowded clinics may not have the time to give their patients the information they need about HIV and AIDS. These patients may not be able to get this information from anywhere else. Free condoms are supplied at clinics. If the clinics are far away, it can be difficult for some people to get the condoms they need.

Illiteracy

Many people who cannot read or write manage their lives very well. But they may not be able to get the information they need to protect themselves against HIV and AIDS.

Unsafe sex

There are many reasons why HIV is spreading to fast. The main reason is that many people have unsafe sex (sex without a condom).

How can you prevent HIV or STDs from spreading?

- You can choose not to have sex at all. If you do not have sex, you are unlikely to get the HIV germ.
- If you do have sex, always have protected sex. Protected sex means that you always use a condom when having sex.
- Only have sex with one partner who you know does not have the HIV germ. The only way to know this is for both of you to be tested for HIV. You and your partner must be faithful to each other after have been tested.
- If you work with blood always wear gloves.
- Clean workplaces with bleach.
- Do not share needles.

Symptoms of AIDS

The symptoms of AIDS are primarily the result of conditions that do not normally develop in individuals with healthy immune systems. Most of these conditions are infections caused by that which are normally controlled by the elements of the immune system that HIV damages, such as:

- bacteria

- viruses

- fungi

- parasites

Opportunistic infections are common in people with AIDS·   These infections affect nearly every organ system.

People with AIDS also have an increased risk of developing various cancers such as Kaposi's sarcoma, cervical cancer and cancers of the immune system known as lymphomas. Additionally, people with AIDS often have systemic symptoms of infection like:

- fevers,

- sweats (particularly at night),

- swollen glands,

- chills,

- weakness, and

- weight loss.

The specific opportunistic infections that AIDS patients develop depend in part on the prevalence of these infections in the geographic area in which the person lives.

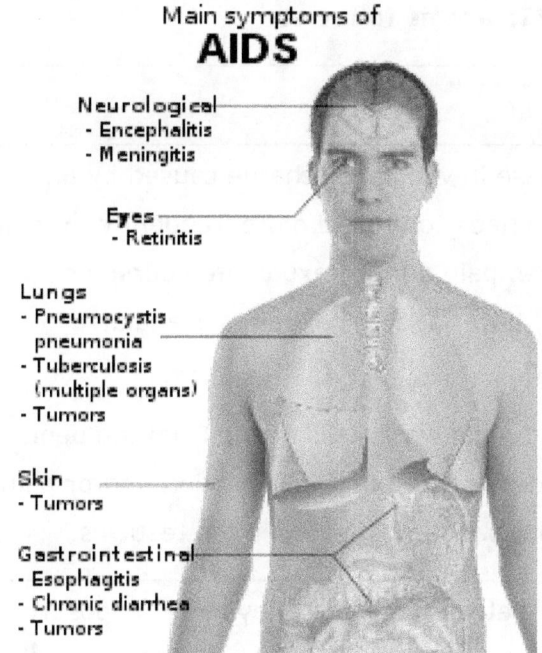

Main symptoms of
AIDS

Neurological
- Encephalitis
- Meningitis

Eyes
- Retinitis

Lungs
- Pneumocystis
  pneumonia
- Tuberculosis
  (multiple organs)
- Tumors

Skin
- Tumors

Gastrointestinal
- Esophagitis
- Chronic diarrhea
- Tumors

Some symptoms in children:

- ○ Wasting syndrome
- ○ Persistent swollen glands
- ○ Recurrent bacterial infections
- ○ Respiratory diseases
- ○ Lymphoid interstitial pneumonia (LIP)
- ○ TB
- ○ Neurological problems
- ○ Skin rashes and skin conditions
- ○ Opportunistic infections

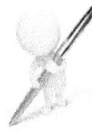

Activity 2:

2.1   Discuss how the HI virus spreads.

2.2   Discuss how one can prevent the HI virus to spread.

2.3   Discuss the symptoms of Aids.

Illnesses that are identified with STDs or STIs are as follows:

STD/STI - Illnesses	Symptoms
Chlamydia	Women: An increase in vaginal discharge caused by an inflamed cervix, he need to urinate more frequently, or pain whilst passing urine, pain during sexual intercourse or bleeding after sex, lower abdominal pains, irregular menstrual bleeding. Men: A white/cloudy and watery discharge from the penis that may stain underwear, a burning sensation and/or pain when passing urine, pain and swelling in the testicles.
Gonorrhea	Symptoms appear between 1 and 14 days after exposure. A burning sensation when urinating, a white/yellow discharge from the penis, a change in vaginal discharge, irritation or discharge from the anus (if the rectum is infected).
Genital Herpes	This will appear 2 to 7 days after first exposure to the virus and last 2 to 4 weeks. Symptoms include itching or tingling sensations in the genital or anal area, small fluid-filled blisters that burst leaving small painful sores, pain when passing urine over the open sores, headaches, backache, flu-like symptoms, including swollen glands or fever.
Genital Warts	The infected person may notice pinkish/white small lumps or larger cauliflower-shaped lumps on the genital area. Genital warts can appear on or around the penis, the scrotum, the thighs or the anus. In women genital warts can develop around the vulva or inside the vagina and on the cervix. If a woman has warts on her cervix, this may cause slight bleeding or, very rarely, an unusual coloured vaginal discharge. Warts may occur singly or in groups. The warts may itch, but they are usually painless.

Syphilis	May take 3 months to appear after sexual contact with an infected person. They include: one or more painless ulcers on the penis, vagina, vulva, cervix, anus or mouth. small lumps in the groin due to swollen glands, a non-itchy rash, fever or flu-like symptoms.
Trichomonas	Discharge in both men and women (sometimes copious and unpleasant smelling in women), discomfort or pain whilst having sex, pain when urinating and inflammation of the urethra.
Bacterial Vaginosis	This may pass unnoticed, it can sometimes produce an abundance of unpleasant fishy smelling discharge.
Crabs	Crabs are lice that can be found in the genital area (as well as other areas) and are noticed around 5 days to 7 weeks after infection and include: itchy skin, inflammation of the affected area, sometimes visible lice and eggs, spots of blood as lice feed from blood vessels in the skin.
Scabies	Symptoms begin 2 to 6 weeks after infection and include: Burrows that appear as silvery or brown wavy lines up to 15 millimetres (half an inch) in length. The burrows can appear anywhere, but usually occur on the webbing between fingers and toes, on the genitals, around the anus, or on the buttocks, elbows or wrists. An intensely itchy rash of inflamed pimple-like lumps (papules/lesions) as an allergic reaction to the mites, their eggs and faeces. Widespread itching, particularly at night or after baths when the body is warmer, as a reaction to the mites.

Misconceptions

A number of misconceptions have arisen surrounding HIV/AIDS. Four of the most common are:

- that AIDS can spread through casual contact,
- that sexual intercourse with a virgin will cure AIDS,
- and that HIV can infect only homosexual men and drug users.
- If the person you want to have sex with looks healthy/is fat you are safe.

Other misconceptions are that any act of anal intercourse between gay men can lead to HIV infection, and that open discussion of homosexuality and HIV in schools will lead to increased rates of homosexuality and AIDS.

Society and Culture

AIDS Stigma exists around the world in a variety of ways including:

- banishment or exclusion,
- social rejection,
- discrimination,
- avoidance of HIV infected people,
- compulsory HIV testing without prior consent or protection of confidentiality,
- violence against HIV infected individuals,
- people who are perceived to be infected with HIV,
- the quarantine of HIV infected individuals.

Stigma-related violence or the fear of violence prevents many people from:

- seeking HIV testing,
- returning for their results,
- or securing treatment.

Turning what could be a manageable chronic illness into a death sentence and perpetuating the spread of HIV.

AIDS stigma has been further divided into the following three categories:

- *Instrumental AIDS stigma*
  A reflection of the fear and apprehension that are likely to be associated with any deadly and transmissible illness.

- *Symbolic AIDS stigma*
  The use of HIV/AIDS to express attitudes toward the social groups or lifestyles perceived to be associated with the disease.

- *Courtesy AIDS stigma*
  Stigmatization of people connected to the issue of HIV/AIDS or HIV- positive people.

Often, AIDS stigma is expressed in conjunction with one or more other stigmas, particularly those associated with:

- homosexuality,

- bisexuality,

- transsexual,

- promiscuity,

- prostitution, and

- intravenous drug use.

In many countries, there is an association between AIDS and homosexuality or bisexuality, and this association is correlated with higher levels of sexual prejudice such as anti-homosexual attitudes. There is also a perceived association between AIDS and all male-male sexual behavior, including sex between uninfected men.

Unfortunately, AIDS discrimination and stigma also fuel the epidemic. They prevent people from talking about their HIV status with sex partners or people with whom they share needles. Fear of rejection and worries about confidentiality also prevent many from getting tested for HIV. This means they may spread HIV to others without knowing it.

How to Cope With AIDS Stigma

There is no simple answer for how to deal with the stigma surrounding HIV and AIDS. The first step might be to seek support from people who understand what you're going through.

- Ask your doctor about local HIV/AIDS support groups. Or, ask to be referred to a psychologist, psychiatrist, or clinical social worker.
- Find a hotline by looking in the yellow pages of your telephone book. Look under "AIDS, HIV Educational Referral and Support Services" or "Social Service Organizations." Ask for practical advice or emotional support over the phone. They can also refer you to local HIV/AIDS self-help organizations.

Examples of AIDS Discrimination

What exactly is AIDS discrimination? It means you are treated differently than other people simply because you are infected with HIV. For example:

- A person denies you access to medical care at a hospital, medical or dental office, skilled nursing facility, or drug treatment centre.
- A person denies you child custody or visitation, or the right to adopt or become a foster parent.
- An employer asks unlawful questions on a job application or harasses, fires, or transfers you to a lesser job position.
- A person of authority reveals your HIV status at school, at work, or within a health care institution.
- You are evicted from a rental property.

Activity 3:

3.1   Discuss the symptoms of 3 STD illnesses.

3.2   Discuss some misconceptions about HIV/Aids.

3.3   Discus the stigma that exists around the world about AIDS.

3.4   Discuss ways in which to cope with Aids stigma.

3.5   Discuss examples of Aids discrimination.

Mother and Child Transmissions

Woman who are HIV positive and pregnant

Women who are HIV positive and pregnant can pass the HIV to their babies. This can be very hard to cope with, especially if you only find out you are HIV positive when you are already pregnant. Women who know that they are HIV positive should think carefully before they decide to have a baby because:

- One out of every three babies born to HIV positive mothers will get HIV if the mother and baby do not take nevirapine to stop this from happening.

- Babies who have the HIV germ get sick often. They usually die when they are very small.

- If you are HIV positive and pregnant, you may get sick with AIDS more quickly.

If you are HIV positive and pregnant, you have the right to terminate the pregnancy. If you chose to do this it is better to have it done early in the pregnancy. An abortion can be done until a woman is 20 weeks pregnant.

> As a HIV positive mother you must live a healthy lifestyle and be careful during your pregnancy so that your baby has the maximum chance of not getting HIV.

Nevirapine is a medicine that lowers the chance of passing HIV to your baby. Your baby must also been given a small amount of Nevirapine within 3 days of birth. Babies take it in syrup form so it is easy for them to swallow. The law says that you and your baby should be treated with Nevirapine if you are HIV positive. Ask the health worker about this.

If you are HIV negative and pregnant you should take precautionary methods not get HIV while you are pregnant by:

- Not having unprotected sex – use a condom at all times,
- Not having sex with different partners.

Your baby can get HIV through:

- Pregnancy
- Birth
- Breastfeeding

Most babies do not live over 8 years who are HIV positive, most die before they are two years old.

Most babies who are HIV positive get sick often. Some of the illnesses will be easy to treat with medicine. A baby who is HIV positive will usually need to go to the clinic or doctor more often than other babies.

Babies who are HIV positive may have some of the following problems:

- Not put on any weight,
- Not grow and develop normally,
- Get diarrhoea a lot,
- Get pneumonia or TB.

It is very painful for parents to see their small baby getting sick so often. It can make them feel helpless and afraid. If your baby is sick, get support.

Breast-feeding and HIV and AIDS

Breast milk is the best food for new babies. It gives them all the goodness they need until they are about six months old. But if you are HIV positive and you breast-feed your baby, there is a chance that you will pass on HIV to your baby during breast-feeding. Here are some things you can do to protect your baby:

- You can squeeze milk from your breasts and boil it well. This will kill HIV and make the milk safe for your baby to drink.
- You can also give your baby milk formula if you can afford it.

HIV/AIDS Testing

Having an HIV test is not an easy decision to make. But the only way to know if one has the HIV germ is to have a blood test.

Why is it important to have the HIV test?

- Having the HIV test means you are taking responsibility for one self.

- It is the only way to know if you are HIV positive or not.

- You need to know how to protect your health. Then you can stay healthy for longer.

- You also need to know how to protect other people from becoming HIV positive.

Having the HIV test

It is important to speak to a counselor or a health worker about having a test. They can help by answering any questions you may have about HIV and AIDS, and about the test.

The counselor knows that you may be afraid and worried about the test or the results. They will give you support, and help you prepare for the results of the test. This is called pre-test counseling.

Some people may choose to take a friend or someone they trust or who has been through the process with them. This person can give them moral support before and after the test.

You will need to talk to a counselor when you go and get your test results. They will discuss the results with you, and what this means. This is called post-test counseling. Remember there are people that care about your wellbeing and want to help and support you throughout this process. You need not be alone in this. Use all the help you can get to get you through the process.

Having the test done

Newer tests can detect the presence of HIV antigen, a protein, up to 20 days earlier than standard tests. This helps prevent spread of the virus to others and start treatment earlier. It is done with a pinprick to the finger.

Here's a look at available HIV tests:

Standard tests	These blood tests check for HIV antibodies. Your body makes antibodies in response to the HIV infection. These tests can't detect HIV in the blood soon after infection because it takes time for your body to make these antibodies. It generally takes two to 8 weeks for your body to produce antibodies, but in some cases it can take up to six months. In standard tests, a small sample of your blood is drawn and sent to a lab for testing. Some of the standard tests use urine or fluids that are collected from the mouth to screen for antibodies.
Rapid antibody tests	Most of these are blood tests for HIV antibodies. Some can detect antibodies in saliva. Results are available in under 30 minutes and are as accurate as standard tests.
Antibody/antigen tests	These tests can detect HIV up to 20 days earlier than standard tests. They check for HIV antigen, a part of the virus that shows up 2-4 weeks after infection. These tests can also detect HIV antibodies. A positive result for the antigen allows treatment to begin earlier and the patient to avoid infecting others. These are blood tests only.
Rapid antibody/antigen test	One antibody/antigen tests delivers results in 20 minutes.
In-home test kits	These kits -- there are two available in the U.S. -- screen blood and saliva for HIV antibodies. You can buy them at your local store. The Home Access HIV-1 Test System requires a small blood sample that is collected at home and sent to a lab. The user, who may remain anonymous, can get results by phone in three business days. The OraQuick In-Home HIV Test can detect HIV antibodies in saliva, if the antibodies are present (which can take up to 6 months). The user swabs the upper and lower gums of their mouths, places the sample in a developer vial, and can get results in 20-40 minutes. A follow-up test should be done if the result is positive.

What if my test is negative?

This means you do not have the HIV germ in your blood. You must still do things:

- You must continue to have protected sex. Do this so that you do not get the germ later.

- If you had unprotected sex recently, the germ may not show up in the first test. Wait for three months and go for another test.

- Continue to learn more about HIV and AIDS.

- Support those in your community who are HIV positive.

What if my test is positive?

When people find out that they are HIV positive they have many strong feelings about it. It is normal to feel angry, hurt and afraid.

It may help to talk to your health worker or a social worker about how you feel. This will help them to feel less alone and afraid.

This is how you may feel when you find out that you are HIV positive:

- Shocked – you may not believe what you hear. You may even deny it and pretend that the results are not correct.
- Angry – you may be angry. You may be angry at yourself because you were not careful enough or had unprotected sex. You may be angry with your partner, and blame them for infecting you.
- Afraid – you may be afraid of how your family will react. You may also be afraid of dying.
- Guilty – you may blame yourself for having unprotected sex.

Always remember that these feelings are normal. There are many ways of trying to deal with your feelings. Learn to be hopeful. Hope gives you the strength to cope with problems. It also helps you to live a normal and healthy life.

Support Groups

Support groups can help people with HIV and AIDS to cope better. If you would like to join a support group, talk to your health worker or else start your own group.

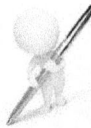

Activity 4:

4.1   Discuss ways how a baby can get HIV/Aids if the mother is infected.

```
_____
_____
_____
```

4.2   Discuss breast feeding and HIV/Aids.

```
_____
_____
_____
```

4.3   Discuss what happens when one goes for an HIV/Aids test.

```
_____
_____
_____
```

4.4   Discuss two different HIV/Aids tests one can take.

```
_____
_____
_____
```

Healthy Life Style

Having HIV AIDS you need to take extra good care of yourself and live a healthy life style. You need to exercise, drink a lot of water, rest and eat healthy.

Healthy food is important for everyone, but especially for HIV positive people. This will help them to be strong, to fight sickness and to stay a healthy weight. Many of the foods we eat everyday are healthy.

HIV positive people should eat as many of these different kinds of food as they can every day.

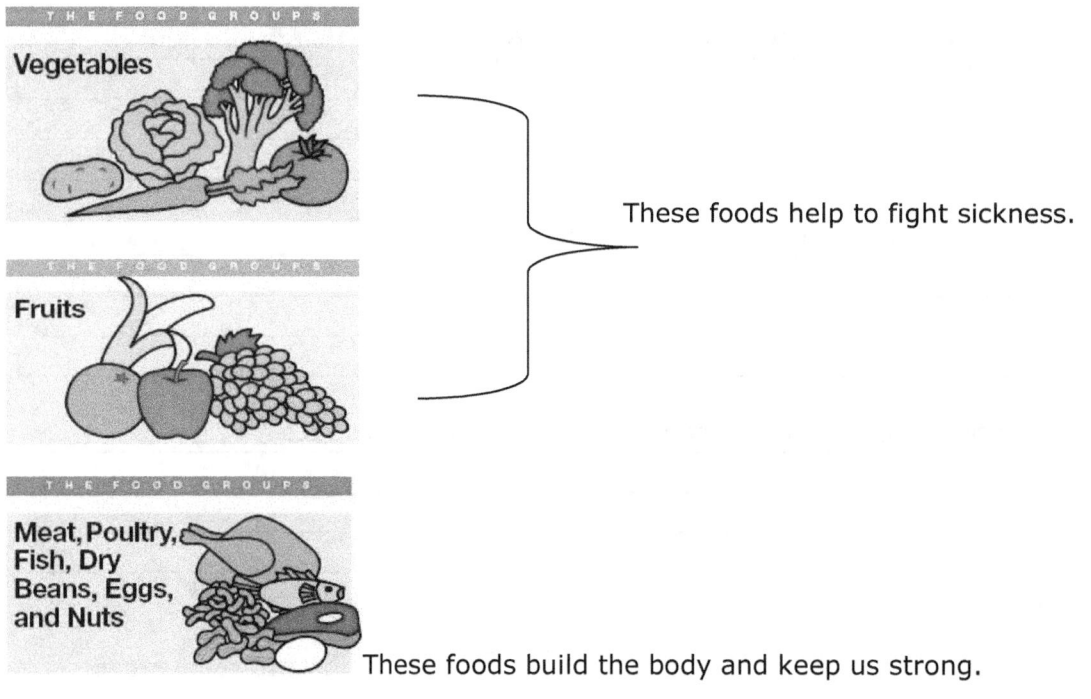

Vegetables

Fruits

These foods help to fight sickness.

Meat, Poultry, Fish, Dry Beans, Eggs, and Nuts

These foods build the body and keep us strong.

Breads, Cereals, Rice, and Pasta

These foods give us energy to grow.

You need to add Butter and oil to your food as this will also provide you with energy.

Prepare and store food safely

If food is not cooked or stored properly, it can carry germs that cause sickness. People who are HIV positive get sick more easily because their immune systems are weaker than other people.

This means it is important to store and cook food properly.

- Cook meat and chicken until there is not pink inside (a clear juice should run from the meat when you cut it open or stick your fork in).

- Do not eat raw pieces of meat. If you are preparing meat do not put your hands in your mouth while touching the meat.

- Clean the services you are going to use to cut your meats or vegetables before and after you prepare your food.

- Do not use cracked eggs or eggs that smell. Boil your eggs for at least 8-10 minutes.

- Heat left-over food to boiling point to kill any germs.

- Wash your hands before and after you prepare or eat food.

- Wash all fruit and vegetables before you eat them.

Healthy eating does not have to be expensive

- Choose vegetables and fruit that are in season as this when they are cheapest. If fruit is too expensive, eat more vegetables.

- Lentils, beans and soya mince are cheaper than meat and chicken.

- Drink water and rooibos tea instead of coffee or fizzy cold drinks.

- Prepare your own fresh food rather than buying meals or take-aways.

- Start your own garden and plant herbs and vegetables for your table (this could be fun as well).

Prevent infections at home

It is not very easy to get HIV when you take care of someone who is HIV positive. But it is important to protect yourself as much as possible.

How to handle dirty washing

- Keep clothes and bedding with blood, diarrhea or body fluids away from other washing.
- Wear plastic bags or gloves on your hands when you work with dirty laundry.
- Wash the bedding and clothes in soapy water. Hang them where there is a lot of sunshine. Make sure washing dries well.
- Bur any bandages that cannot be rewashed.
- Do not touch body fluids such as blood, stool and urine. Wear plastic bags or gloves on your hands when you clean a sick person.
- Wash the gloves or plastic bags in hot water every time after you have used them.
- Do not share needles, razors or toothbrushes.
- Keep all sores clean and covered. Make sure everyone in the home does this.

How to keep the bed clean

It is important to keep the sick person's mattress, sheets, blankets and pillows clean. Do this by covering the mattress with a plastic sheet.

You can make your own plastic sheet by ironing big plastic bags together. Make sure that you use strong bags, like the 12KG plastic mielie-meal bags.

Wash the sheets, blankets and pillows as often as you can. Wipe the plastic sheet with a hot, wet cloth.

Living Positively

It is true that there is no cure for HIV AIDS. But that does not mean that you cannot live a happy life. You could live positively with the sickness. You can still live a quality life and if you take good care of yourself you could still live quite long life. To live positively with HIV and AIDS means:

- You can live with hope.

- You can share your life with family and friends.

- You can make a positive impact on other people's lives.

- You can talk about your problems.

- You can live a healthy life with enough exercise and rest.

- You can eat healthy food.

- Try to work for a long as possible.

Remember that people with HIV/Aids are still alive, and that they can still enjoy their life.

Some points of taking care of your mind and body

- Although food will not cure HIV, but it can help to keep your immune system strong. Eat fresh food like fruit and vegetables, beans, chicken and fish.

- Stop smoking and drinking as this makes your body week. It is then easier for HIV to attack your body and for you to get AIDS earlier.

- Join a support group of people living with HIV and ADS. Talk to someone when you feel lonely, sad or angry.

- Go for regular checkups (every 3-4 months). Your health worker will give you advice, and will help you to deal with any problems you have.

- Treat any new diseases or problems:

  o It is important to go to the clinic if you are sick. This is because every sickness makes your body weaker and less able to fight HIV.

  o If the clinic finds that you have any new sickness or problems, they should treat them.

  o If these sicknesses are not treated quickly, they may get worse and make you very sick.

Anti-retroviral medicines:

- There are some medicines that can slow down HIV and keep you well for a long time.
- These medicines are very expensive and need to be taken every day, month after month and year after year.
- Talk to the health worker about these medicines.

Advances in HIV Treatment: Understanding ART

Antiretroviral therapy -- or ART -- revolutionized HIV treatment in the past few decades. And newer improvements, like one-pill-a-day drugs, are making life with HIV easier and safer.

"HIV really is a chronic disease now," says Brad Hare, MD, medical director of the HIV/AIDS Division at San Francisco General Hospital. "It's like diabetes or high blood pressure." As long as you manage it well, you should expect a long, healthy life.

Understanding ART

ART works by combining drugs that attack the virus in different ways. ART doesn't cure HIV. But it stops it from reproducing itself and spreading.

Doctors measure HIV by the viral load -- that's the amount of the virus that's in your bloodstream. The goal of treatment is to get the viral load so low that tests can't even detect the virus anymore. HIV is still there, but there's not enough of it to cause symptoms -- as long as you keep taking your medication. Also remember that you can still pass HIV to someone else while on medication.

5 Things to Know About HIV Medications

There are lots of myths and stale, outdated information about HIV treatment. Here are five things you should know about ART.

- **It's easier to take than it used to be.** A lot of people with HIV just take one pill once a day. That's it. That one combination pill -- Atripla, Complera, or Stribild -- packs in all the different active ingredients you need. Most people don't need the "cocktails" with complicated dosing schedules anymore.
- **You have lots of options.** Some people need drug combinations. There are six classes of antiretroviral drugs for HIV and more than 30 drugs. If one doesn't work or causes side effects, the doctor has many other choices.
- **Medications work for a long time.** People used to worry that their drugs would stop working after a while and that they'd have to keep switching to new ones. That's not really a risk now. "As long as you keep taking your medications, the same treatment can work for decades," Hare says.
- **Drugs have fewer side effects.** While specific side effects depend on the drug, HIV treatment is much safer and easier to tolerate than it used to be. For most people, side effects -- like upset stomach and diarrhoea -- are minor and often go away. Long-term risks include cholesterol problems and weakened bones. But even so, the risks of treatment are much lower than the risks of not getting it, Hare says.
- **You may start taking medication as soon as you're diagnosed.** Many experts believe that the sooner you start treatment, the better. However, some doctors prefer to wait until your CD4 count, a measure of some immune cells, drops to a certain point before starting treatment. See what your doctor recommends.

The Groups of Antiretroviral Drugs

There are four main groups of anti-HIV drugs, however, as research continues new classes of drugs are continually being added in the fight against HIV and AIDS. Each of these groups attacks HIV in a different way.

Nucleoside Reverse Transcriptase Inhibitors: The first group of antiretroviral drugs are the Nucleoside Reverse Transcriptase Inhibitors (NRTIs). They were the first type of drug available to treat HIV infection in 1987 and are better known as nucleoside analogues or nukes. HIV needs an enzyme called reverse transcriptase in order to be able to infect healthy cells and reproduce itself in a person's body. As the name says, NRTIs inhibit reverse transcriptase. The drugs slow down the production of the reverse transcriptase enzyme and make HIV unable to infect cells and duplicate itself.

Non-Nucleoside Reverse Transcriptase Inhibitors: The second group of antiretroviral drugs are the Non-Nucleoside Reverse Transcriptase Inhibitors (NNRTIs). These drugs started to be approved in 1997 and are generally referred as non-nucleosides or non-nukes. This group of drugs also stops HIV from infecting cells by intervening with the trancriptase of the virus. The non-nucleoside drugs work slightly differently from the nucleoside analogues in that they bind in a different way to the cell's reverse transcriptase. The non-nucleoside drugs block the duplication and the spread of HIV.

Protease Inhibitors: The third type of antiretrovirals is the Protease Inhibitor (PI) group. They were first approved in 1995. Protease inhibitors, as the name says, inhibit protease. Almost every living cell contains protease. Protease is a digestive enzyme that breaks down protein and is one of the many enzymes that HIV uses to reproduce itself.

The protease in HIV attacks the long healthy chains of enzymes and proteins in the cells and cuts them into smaller pieces. These infected smaller pieces of proteins and enzymes continue to infect new cells. The protease inhibitors take effect before the protease in HIV has the chance to break down the protein and enzymes. This way the protease inhibitors slow down the duplication of the virus and thus prevent the infection of new cells. The NRTIs and NNRTIs only have an effect on newly infected cells. Protease inhibitors are able to slow the process of immature non-infectious virus becoming mature and infectious. Protease inhibitors also work in cells that have been infected for a long time, by slowing down the reproduction of the virus.

Fusion or Entry Inhibitors: The fourth group of antiretrovirals are called Fusion or Entry Inhibitors. The first of these drugs (Fuzeon) has recently been approved. The surface of HIV carries proteins called gp41 and gp120. These are the proteins which allow HIV to attach itself to and enter into cells. By blocking one of these proteins, fusion inhibitors slow down the reproduction of the virus. For example, Fuzeon sticks to the protein gp41. Fuzeon differs from the other antiretrovirals in that it needs to be injected. It is a protein and cannot be taken orally, since it would be digested in the stomach. [*This copyrighted article is courtesy of AVERT*]

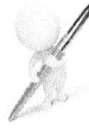

Activity 5:

5.1　Discuss how one can live healthy even if you have obtained HIV/Aids.

5.2　Discuss the advances in HIV/Aids treatments.

5.3　Discuss two types of drugs used for the treatment of HIV/Aids.

Your Rights and Responsibilities

You have the right to:

1. Be listened to.
2. Say what you feel and think in a respectful manner.
3. Say "no" to something you don't want to do or don't believe in, without feeling guilty.
4. Say "I need time to think about that."

Each of us has the responsibility to acknowledge the concerns of others and negotiate to resolve our differences.

Should I have sex?"

A simple question with no simple answer, right?

Only **you know** if you're really ready. If you're not sure, we're here to help you decide.

Ask yourself, would you have sex if you:

- Didn't know enough about your partner?
- Couldn't predict how having sex would affect your relationship?
- Didn't know enough about preventing pregnancy and sexually transmitted infections (STIs)?

There are many pathways to choose from when it comes to having sex. Communicating, dating and relationship issues, and other ways to be intimate all play a part in deciding whether you should or shouldn't have sex.

But no matter the path, in the end you'll reach one of two possible destinations: gladness or regret.

Remember the decision lies with you always. Nobody may force you into something you do not want to do. If they do – they do not really love you. You would not want to be in a relationship where you are not respected and where you have no rights to make decisions for yourself anyway.

Quiz – Should you or shouldn't you?

This brief quiz asks you to answer important questions about your knowledge, values and feelings about having sex. Answering each question truthfully will help you decide.

When you've finished the quiz, ask your partner to take it too.

		Yes	No
1	Do both my partner and I feel ready to have sex now?	○	○
2	Have my partner and I talked about what having sex means to our relationship?	○	○
3	Do I know my reasons for deciding to have sex now?	○	○
4	Will I feel good about myself if I have sex now?	○	○
5	Am I sure no one is pressuring me to have sex?	○	○
6	Can I say "No" to sex without feeling guilty?	○	○
7	Can my partner and I openly discuss the prevention of sexually transmitted infections and pregnancy?	○	○
8	Does my partner and I know enough about how to prevent sexually transmitted infections and pregnancy?	○	○
9	Are we responsible enough to use condoms and a method of birth control every time we have sex?	○	○
10	Are we ready to handle the possible consequences of being sexually active?	○	○
11	If the relationship breaks up, will I regret having had sex with this person?	○	○

If either of you answered "NO" to any question, now is probably NOT the right time for you.

Be Assertive, Not Aggressive when saying NO!

People often think they're being *assertive* when in fact they're being aggressive. But they're not the same.

You're being *aggressive* when:

- You're being hostile or blaming someone.
- You threaten or demand.
- You use sarcasm to try to make your point.
- Your behaviour and comments are disrespectful to not only your feelings and rights, but also the feelings and rights of others.

You're being *assertive* when:

- You clearly express your feelings and your rights.
- You speak and act in your own best interests but still consider the needs and rights of others.
- You develop trust and equality in your relationships.
- You ask for help when you need it.

How to Be Assertive

You can learn to be assertive using three steps. (These steps will start to blend together and sound more natural the more you practice.)

Let's say you agree to pick up your partner in the morning before classes – your partner is always late which makes you late for your morning classes. What should you do?

STEP 1: Describe the Situation

Describe what happened. Give only the facts.
"Since I have started picking you up to go to school, I am late for my morning classes".

STEP 2: State How You Feel

Tell the person how their behaviour or action makes you feel (i.e., sad, angry or afraid) and why.

"I feel anxious and frustrated when I am late for class. I feel I am being disrespectful when I walk into class late".

STEP 3: State What You Need

Describe the action you need to see and a promise or commitment that it will happen.
"I need you to be on time in the mornings so I am not late".

Tips

- Always remember to use "I want" or "I feel" statements. Saying "I want" instead of "You are" will keep you focused on your own feelings.
- Try lowering the tension with humour. Lighten the tone of your voice and smile as you make your point.
- Being assertive isn't just for problem situations. Use these steps to compliment, support, and encourage someone you care about.

Being assertive when your partner does not want to use a condom is very important. The bottom line is "no sex without a condom".

Here are some tips to help you talk to your partner about safe sex:

Your partner says: "We have not used a condom before. Why do you want to use a condom now?

You can reply: "Now I know more about HIV and Aids. We have not had an HIV test. We do not know whether we are carrying HIV. That is why I think we should use a condom."

Your partner says: "I cannot feel anything when we use a condom."

You can reply: "Try it! I'm sure you will still feel a lot."

Your partner says: "I don't feel sick. And I am careful about who I have sex with."

You can reply: "I don't feel sick either. But we have not had an HIV test, so we could both have HIV and not know it."

Activity 6:

6.1   Explain your rights with regards to protecting yourself against HIV/Aids.

6.2   Explain what it means to be assertive.

6.3   What should you be asking yourself whether or not to have sex?

SECTION 2 – HEALTH AND SAFETY AWARENESS

Course Overview

Workplace accidents and injuries cost corporations millions of dollars and thousands of hours lost every year. They also have a profound, often lifelong impact on workers. Introducing a safety culture into your organization, where safety is valued as an integral part of the business' operation, not only saves the business time and money, it also builds a committed, loyal, healthy workforce. This section will give you the foundation to start building your safety culture.

Course Overview

After you have completed this section you will be able to:

- Understand the difference between a safety program and a safety culture.
- Have some resources to help you understand the regulations in your area.
- Be able to launch a safety committee.
- Understand how to identify hazards and reduce them.
- Know some hiring measures that can improve safety.
- Understand what a safety training program will involve.
- Be able to identify groups particularly at risk for injury and know how to protect them.
- Be able to help your organization write, implement, and review a safety plan.
- Be better able to respond to incidents and near misses.
- Understand the basics of accident investigation and documentation.
- Discuss and explain the purpose of safety equipment and procedures.

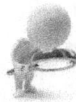

Go through the following table, this is an indication of what you will be expected to know and demonstrate an understanding in. Once you have completed this course return to this section and assess whether you grasp each specific outcome.

Specific Outcome	Assessment Criteria	Yes	No
1. Identify potential hazards in the work area.	• I am able to identify potential hazards correctly and removed, reduced or reported. • I am able to explain implications of exposure to hazardous substances and hazards. • I am able to draw up health and safety plans. • I am able to identify protective clothing requirements and where necessary protective clothing is used. • I am able to demonstrate that all statutory requirements are being met.		
2. Limit damage to persons or property in the case of an emergency.	• I am able to identify the location of fire extinguishers, hoses and alarms. • I am able to identify different fire extinguishers and is used correctly. • I am able to identify procedures of emergencies are known and followed promptly and correctly. • I am able to report injuries involving individuals promptly to the relevant persons.		
3. Follow procedures that apply to illness or injury in the work area.	• I am able to explain procedures for reporting and recording are demonstrated. • I am able to explain procedures to be followed if an injury may lead to a claim against workman's compensation are followed. • I am able to explain a brief incident report is written and delivered to the relevant authority.		
4. Essential Embedded Knowledge.	• I am able to explain "hazard", "hazardous substance", "risk" and "safe" as described in the Occupational Health & Safety Act (Act no. 85 of 1993), and the relationship between the three concepts. • I am able to explain Statutory requirements. • I am able to explain Workman`s compensation procedures. • I am able to explain Relevant national regulations. • I am able to explain Health and safety regulations. • I am able to explain The implications of not following procedure that apply to illness or injury in the work area. • I am able to explain Health and safety planning. • I am able to explain the use of protective clothing. • I am able to explain the use of fire extinguishers. • I am able to explain procedures for incident reporting and recording.		

Safety should not be viewed as a single program, a quick fix, or an overnight project. In order for your workplace to be truly safe, safety must be part of you're and your organization's culture and value system.

How Does Safety Apply to Me?

When you think of the need for a safety culture, you probably think of high-risk environments like factories and construction sites. However, regardless of your organization's industry, you do need to be concerned about safety.

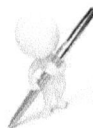

Activity 7: Discuss the following situations and what safety issues could occur?

Situation	Safety Issues
Insurance office with four people, each in their own cubicle (equipped with computer and telephone).	
Animal rescue facility.	
Medical transcriptionists that work from home.	

Do you have other unique examples of situations where we must be conscious of safety?

Your employer will make every effort to ensure the health and safety of their staff is adhered to under the Occupational Health and Safety Act (OHS Act).

DUTIES OF THE EMPLOYER

OHS Act Section 8 General Duties of Employer to their Employees

(1) Every employer shall provide and maintain, as far as is reasonably practicable, a working environment that is safe and without risk to the health of his employees.

(2) Without derogating from the generality of an employer's duties under subsection (1), the matters to which those duties refer include in particular-

    (a) the provision and maintenance of systems of work, plant and machinery that, as far as is reasonably practicable, are safe and without risks to health;

    (b) taking such steps as may be reasonably practicable to eliminate or mitigate any hazard or potential hazard to the safety or health of employees, before resorting to personal protective equipment;

    (c) making arrangements for ensuring, as far as is reasonably practicable, the safety and absence of risks to health in connection with the production, processing, use, handling, storage or transport of articles or substances;

    (d) establishing, as far as is reasonably practicable, what hazards to the health or safety of persons are attached to any work which is performed, any article or substance which is produced, processed, used, handled, stored or transported and any plant or machinery which is used in his business, and he shall, as far as is reasonably practicable, further establish what precautionary measures should be taken with respect to such work, article, substance, plant or machinery in order to protect the health and safety of persons, and he shall provide the necessary means to apply such precautionary measures;

    (e) providing such information, instructions, training and supervision as may be necessary to ensure, as far as is reasonably practicable, the health and safety at work of his employees;

    (f) as far as is reasonably practicable, not permitting any employee to do any work or to produce, process, use, handle, store or transport any article or substance or to operate any plant or machinery, unless the precautionary measures contemplated in paragraphs (b) and (d), or any other precautionary measures which may be prescribed, have been taken;

    (g) taking all necessary measures to ensure that tire requirements of this Act are complied with by every person in his employment or on premises under his control where plant or machinery is used;

    (h) enforcing such measures as may be necessary in the interest of health and safety;

(i)   ensuring that work is performed and that plant or machinery is used under the general supervision of a person trained to understand the hazards associated with it and who have the authority to ensure that precautionary measures taken by the employer are implemented; and

(j)   causing all employees to be informed regarding the scope of their authority as contemplated in section 37 (1) (b).

OHS Act Section 9   **General Duties of Employers and Self Employed Persons to persons other than their employees**

(1) Every employer shall conduct his understanding in such a way as to ensure, as far as is reasonably practicable, that persons other than those in his employment who may be directly affected by his activities are not thereby exposed to hazards to their health or safety.

(2) Every self-employed person shall conduct his undertaking in such a manner as to ensure, as far as is reasonably practicable, that he and other persons who may be directly affected by his activities are not thereby exposed to hazards to their health or safety.

OHS Act Section 16   **Chief Executive Officer Charged with certain duties**

(1) Every chief executive officer shall as far as reasonably practicable ensure that the duties of his employer as contemplated in this Act, are properly discharged.

(2) Without derogating from his responsibility or liability in terms of subsection (1), a chief executive officer may assign any duty contemplated in the said subsection, to any person under his control, which person shall act subject to the control and directions of the chief executive officer.

(3) The provisions of subsection (1) shall not, subject to the provisions of section 37, relieve an employer or any responsibility or any liability under this Act.

(4) For the purpose of subsection (1), the head of department of any department of State shall be deemed to be the chief executive officer of that department.

DUTIES OF THE EMPLOYEE

OHS Act Section 14   **General duties of employees at work**

Every employee shall at work-

(a)   take reasonable care for the health and safety of himself and of other persons who may be affected by his acts or omissions;

(b)   as regards any duty or requirement imposed on his employer or any other person by this Act, co-operate with such employer or person to enable that duty or requirement to be performed or complied with;

(c)   carry out any lawful order given to him, and obey the health and safety rules and procedures laid down by his employer or by anyone authorized thereto by his employer, in the interest of health or safety;

(d)   if any situation which is unsafe or unhealthy comes to his attention, as soon as practicable report such situation to his employer or to the health and safety representative for his workplace or section thereof, as the case may be, who shall report it to the employer; and

(e)   if he is involved in any incident which may affect his health or which has caused an injury to himself, report such incident to his employer or to anyone authorized thereto by the employer, or to his health and safety representative, as soon as practicable but not later than the end of the particular shift during which the incident occurred, unless the circumstances were such that the reporting of the incident was not possible, in which case he shall report the incident as soon as practicable thereafter.

There are various regulations under the Act which might affect your company and you are advised to familiarize yourself with this.

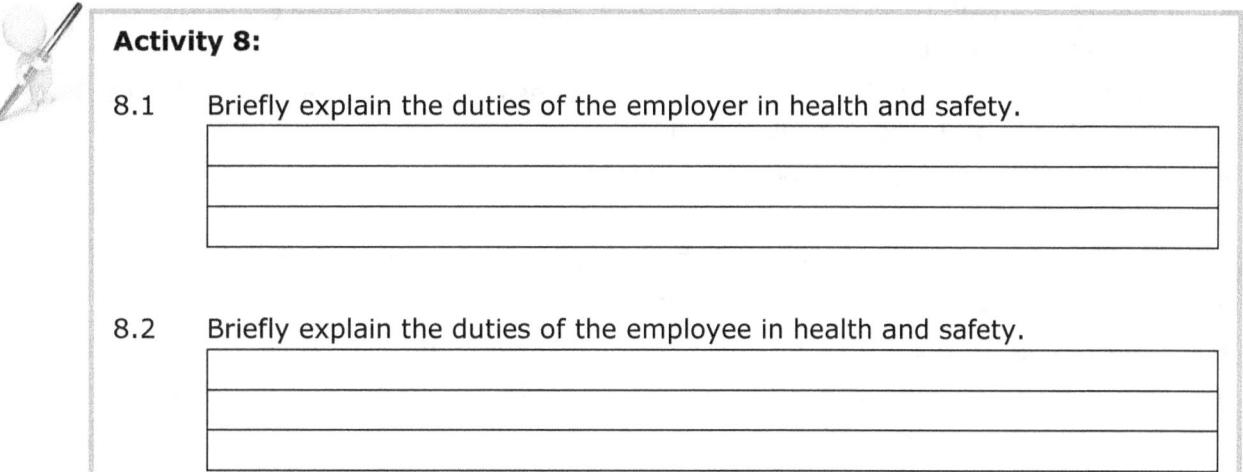

Activity 8:

8.1   Briefly explain the duties of the employer in health and safety.

8.2   Briefly explain the duties of the employee in health and safety.

Remember the following to help you comply with the regulations:

- Appoint a Health and Safety representative to form a workplace committee.
- Ensure you have first aid facilities such as first aid boxes and trained personnel to act as first aiders.
- Establish emergency procedures and communicate these to staff and visitors.
- Have regular fire drills – minimal Legal Requirement is yearly.
- Keep a record of who is in the workplace at any time, in case of fire.
- Fire exits must be clearly marked with regulatory green signage.
- Never block fire exits, escape routes or fire fighting equipment.
- Have an evacuation plan and assembly point where a roll call will be held.
- Ensure you have the correct type and amount of fire fighting equipment for the size of your building. This must be checked monthly and a record (Register) kept. Fire extinguishers should be serviced on a yearly basis by a Accredited Service Provider. Failure to do this could result in your insurance company refusing to pay you in the event of a claim!
- Conduct fire training including evacuation procedure and use of equipment at least every 3 years or when need is required.
- Store all hazardous materials in a safe place and as per legislation.
- Know the telephone number of the fire brigade, ambulance service, poison centre and police.
- Hold regular safety meetings for staff to identify hazards and areas for improvement.
- Wilful violation of health and safety regulations by an employer or employee is a serious criminal offence and punishable by law (Section 38 of the OHS Act).
- Set up a procedure whereby hazards are reported immediately by your employees and the appropriate action is taken.
- Ensure that staff is careful around machinery and don't wear loose clothing and jewellery when operating machinery.
- Make sure that staff always observes instructions for machinery and are fully trained in the safe use of the equipment / machines.
- All accidents need to be reported immediately or as soon as possible but before the end of their shift.
- Make sure employees always wear the necessary protective clothing.
- Smoking regulations must be observed at all times.
- Spilled objects must be cleaned up immediately as per the Chemical Spills Procedure.
- Work areas should be kept clean and tidy and rubbish should be disposed of regularly.

Main features of OHS Act
- Regulating health and hygiene in addition to safety.
- The employer's duty to provide information, training and supervision.
- The election of HSE Representatives and the establishing of health and safety committees.
- The employer's duty to prevent an accident prior to taking corrective actions.
- Severe penalties for failing to maintain a healthy and safe workplace.

The Act creates a standard

- The Act sets out legal rules and penalties, which creates a standard that everyone can be aware of. Without such a standard, all reasonable employees would have their own approach to health and safety and this obviously would lead to confusion.

If there were no Act

- "Absolute safety under all circumstances is not guaranteed to the labourer by the contract of employment. The employer is not an insurer. **He is not bound to furnish the safety machinery, nor to provide the best possible means of its operation** in order to relieve him from responsibility".   (Union Government vs Barker)

Creating a Safety Committee

There are several key steps to creating a safety committee.

- A health and safety committee will be established according to the size of the organisation and the number of health and safety representatives.
- All health and safety representatives shall be members of the committee.
- In the case of shift work, at least one health and safety representative for that specific workplace shall attend the meeting.

An executive health and safety committee may also be established or at least health and safety are to be on the agenda as a discussion point at management meeting.

Health and Safety Committees

- OHS Act places a duty on the employer to establish at least one H&S Committee where two or more representatives have been appointed.
- They can hold meetings as often as necessary, although the minimum requirements are once every three months.

Members of Committee

- **Employee representatives** (Health and Safety Representatives)
- **Employer Representatives** (Should not exceed the no. of H&S reps)
- **Co-opted / Advisory Members** (No voting power)

Measures

At every meeting the employer shall consult with the committee regarding the following measures to ensure OH&S at the workplace:

- Initiating measures,
- Developing measures,
- Promoting measures,
- Monitoring and reviewing measures.

Evaluating the effectiveness of meetings

- Were there objectives?
- Were the objectives achieved?
- Were all the members present?
- Did they make significant contributions?
- Were the items on the agenda concise?
- Was the meeting planned thoroughly and was it convenient as far as venue, date and time?

Functions of OH&S Committees

- Discuss health and safety representative reports,
- Discuss incident investigation reports,
- Discuss potential hazards reported to committee,
- Discuss employee complaints,
- Investigate incidents / accidents,
- Make recommendations on all above and consult with the employer regarding c/a.

Health and Safety Representatives

- Only those employees employed in full time capacity at a specific workplace, who is literate i.e. can read and write and who are acquainted with the specific working conditions and activities at the workplace shall be eligible for appointment as health and safety representative for that specific workplace.
- At least one health and safety representative for every 50 employees in operation and one for every 100 employees in offices shall be nominated / elected / appointed and trained after consultation between management and their employees and / or representatives.
- Health and safety representatives, once nominated and elected will be appointed in writing for a specific workplace / constituency and for a period of two years. The health and safety representative must acknowledge their acceptance of the appointment letter. A transfer from the appointed area or written requisition will terminate the appointment of a health and safety representative.
- A health and safety representative who does not perform the duties / functions assigned to him / her, will be requested in writing by the health and safety committee to perform these duties within 10 working days. Should the health and safety representative fail to respond to this instruction, his / her appointment will be withdrawn and nominations will be asked within the constituency to replace the health and safety representative.

Functions / Obligations

Apart from the functions of a health and safety representative as per OHS Act, he / she will be required to:

- Make personal contact monthly with all employees he / she represents and record their concerns in his / her inspection register.
- Make representation regarding health and safety issues to management through the health and safety committee for the workplace he / she represents.
- Health and safety representative will receive training during working hours.
- Health and safety representative will be allowed to conduct inspections during working hours within his designated area of responsibility, provided that prior notice is given to his appointed supervisor or Head of department.
- Health and safety representatives must obtain permission from their respective supervisors / Head of Department prior to leaving their workplaces to perform their functions. Such permission shall not be unreasonably withheld.

Functions of Health and Safety Reps

A health and safety rep. **May and shall be Entitled** to:

- The health and safety representative has numerous functions and these functions must be carried out during normal working hours and without additional remuneration.

Their main functions are:

- Inspections,
- Accident investigations,
- Committee meetings,
- Personal contacts with employees.

Health and Safety Representative Inspections

- Know what to look for,
- Practice inspections,
- Keep an open mind,
- Beware of general impressions,
- Guard against the habit of familiarity,
- Make personal contact and TALK TO PEOPLE,
- Record findings.

Seven ways to kill Health and Safety Representatives

- Responsibility and Accountability no Authority,
- Negative assigned persons, Section 16(2) or 8(2)(1),
- No dynamic OH&S committees,
- Not involved in accident investigations,
- No feedback on decisions taken,

- No management support,
- No ownership.

Provide resources

Make the safety committee's job as easy as possible. Provide them with whatever resources they need to start developing a safety culture in organization. This may include training, resource materials, or perhaps just a comfortable place to meet.

The Safety Committee's First Meeting

An agenda should be circulated beforehand and presented at the beginning of the meeting. The meeting should also start on time to set a good precedent for future meetings.

Example of a Health and Safety Committee Agenda.

9:00-9:10	Introductions.
9:10-9:30	Briefing by Tammy Smith, CEO. (To discuss the desired scope and mission of the safety committee)
9:30-9:45	Setting of team norms . (These are ground rules that the team will agree to conduct meetings by, such as "Managers will leave their manager hat at the door," or, "We will listen to each other's opinions.")
9:45-10:00	Team name and mission; election of chairperson and minute taker.
10:00-10:30	Identification of tasks and actions to be taken.
10:45-11:00	Time, place, and agenda for future meetings.

The Hazard Identification Process

Identifying hazards is a key step in making the workplace safer. This is a task that the safety committee can take on, with the assistance of all employees in the workforce.

There are several key ways to identify hazards.

Look at accident reports

Review past accidents and near misses. List the key facts of the incidents and look for patterns.

Perform a job safety analysis. (Internal Risk Assessment)

Although this can be time-consuming, it is the best way to identify hazards. With this method, you review each job. You look at each task that the job entails and the method used to perform each task. Then, review each step for possible hazards. (A good way to test the safety of the step is to think, "Would I want my child doing this task this way?")

Ideally, this analysis will be performed with the employee to ensure every possible hazard is identified.

Use a checklist

A checklist can help organize the walkthrough, ensure that nothing is missed. It can also help identify common industry hazards. However, it may be too comprehensive or it could exclude aspects particular to your workplace. If you're going to use a checklist, have the safety committee review it first to ensure that it is applicable and appropriate.

Example: Health and Safety Checklist

HSE REPRESENTATIVE INSPECTION REGISTER

Department: _____   Month: _____

HSE Rep Name: _____   Year: _____

		Inspection Criteria	Deviation identified
1.		Building and floors clean and in good condition.	
2.		Housekeeping of good standard.	
3.		Workplace tidy & clear of material and equipment not used.	
4.		Stacking and storage safe, available storage space well used.	
5.		Demarcation visible and complied with.	
6.		Lighting level sufficient, no lights out, windows clean.	
7.		Sufficient ventilation, fresh air, air movement.	
8.		Pollution of ground, water, air prevented.	
9		Yard tidy and clear of waste and material and equipment not used.	
10.		Sufficient and correct type of waste bins available and frequently emptied.	
11.		Colour coding in place: pipes, machines & switches.	
12.		Portable electrical equipment numbered, on register and inspected to ensure safe condition for use.	
13.		Machine guarding in place.	
14.		Lock-out system in place and used.	
15.		Electrical switches labelled/numbered.	
16.		Signage risk related and in place.	
17.		Ladders in good condition, on register and inspected.	
18.		Ladders stored appropriately.	
19.		Scaffolding proper storage and inspected before use.	
20.		Lifting gear: in good condition,	
	•	properly used,	
	•	operator licensed where necessary,	
	•	on maintenance register.	
21.		Compressed gasses: cylinders used correctly and safely	
	•	cylinders safely stored/chained.	
22.		Gas welding sets on register and inspected	
23.		Hazardous chemical substances: safely stored	
	•	containers labelled.	
	•	data on chemicals available in work area.	
	•	correct PPE worn when chemicals are used.	
	•	transported as per SABS codes.	
24.		Motorised vehicles, forklifts and trolleys numbered, on register and inspected.	
25.		Hand tools inspected, kept clean and in good working order.	
26.		Safety belt and harnesses numbered, on register and inspected.	
27.		Eye protection: issued and worn correctly where indicated	

	• eye protection kept clean and stored correctly.	
28.	Foot protection: issued and worn correctly where indicated.	
	• foot protection is kept clean and is in good condition.	
29.	Hearing protection: issued and worn correctly where indicated	
	• hearing protection clean and in good condition.	
	• hearing zones are clearly demarcated.	
30.	Hand protection: issued and worn where indicated	
	• correct hand protection is used.	
	• hand protection clean and stored correctly.	
	• hand protection disposed of correctly.	
	• hand protection replaced when necessary.	
31.	Respirators: correct type issued and worn correctly where indicated	
	• respirators kept clean and stored correctly.	
	• record kept of cleaning and maintenance.	
	• worn respirators disposed of correctly.	
32.	Inspection of PPE is done.	
33.	Fire equipment: in place	
	• equipment numbered.	
	• seals intact.	
	• signage in place and visible.	
	• demarcation visible and complied with.	
	• fire fighters trained and available in area.	
	• emergency plan communicated to staff members.	
	• emergency evacuation plan displayed.	
34.	Emergency plan available in case of chemical spillage.	
35.	Safety notice board kept neat and up to date.	
36.	Safety Policy communicated and displayed.	
37.	HSE incidents reported to appropriate persons.	
38.	First aid box in place, identified, inspected and kept up to date.	
39.	Trained first aiders available in area.	
40.	Waste minimization practices in place.	
41.	Recycling done where possible.	
42.	Resource conservation in place where possible.	
43.	HSE risks are communicated to staff members.	
44.	Hazards related to tasks are communicated to staff members before task is performed.	
45	Feedback from HSE committee meeting is given to staff members.	

ADDITIONAL ITEMS INSPECTED

	Item inspected	Deviation identified
46.		
47.		
48.		
49.		
50.		
51.		
52.		

GENERAL REMARKS

DEVIATIONS AND HAZARDS REPORTED

No	Description	Corrective Action	Date complete

HEALTH, SAFETY AND ENVIRONMENTAL REPRESENTATIVE

Remarks:

Signature	Date

HEALTH, SAFETY & ENVIRONMENTAL CO-ORDINATOR

Remarks:

Signature	Date

HEALTH, SAFETY & ENVIRONMENTAL COMMITTEE

This report was discussed by this committee at the meeting held on _____ at _____ and the following comments were made:

Signature of Chairperson	Date

EMPLOYER

Remarks:

Signature of Employer	Date

or Assigned Person

Review Hazards

It is important to note that hazards should be reviewed at a pre-determined interval. Other events that may trigger hazard re-identification can include:

- Addition of new equipment,
- Office re-location,
- Change in job responsibilities,
- New pattern of incidents,
- Issue raised by staff member.

Common Hazards

Hazards will differ from workplace to workplace as there are so many variables to consider. However, here are some of the most common types of hazards.

Area	Description
Health	Extreme temperatures, air quality , noise.
Biological	Exposure to illnesses, sick buildings. (i.e., those with mold or toxins)
Chemical	Toxic substances. (gases, solids, or liquids)
Ergonomical	Activities that can cause repetitive strain injuries.
Physical	Physical elements of the workplace, including lighting, floors, ceilings, stairs, ramps, and machinery.

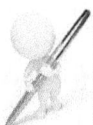

Hazard Identification for the Acme Widget Company

You have been assigned an important job: evaluating possible hazards at the Acme Widget Company. Take a look at the information provided below and identify some hazards.

Part One: Case Study

The Acme Widget Company manufactures and distributes widgets. It occupies the main floor of a warehouse. The floor plan looks like this:

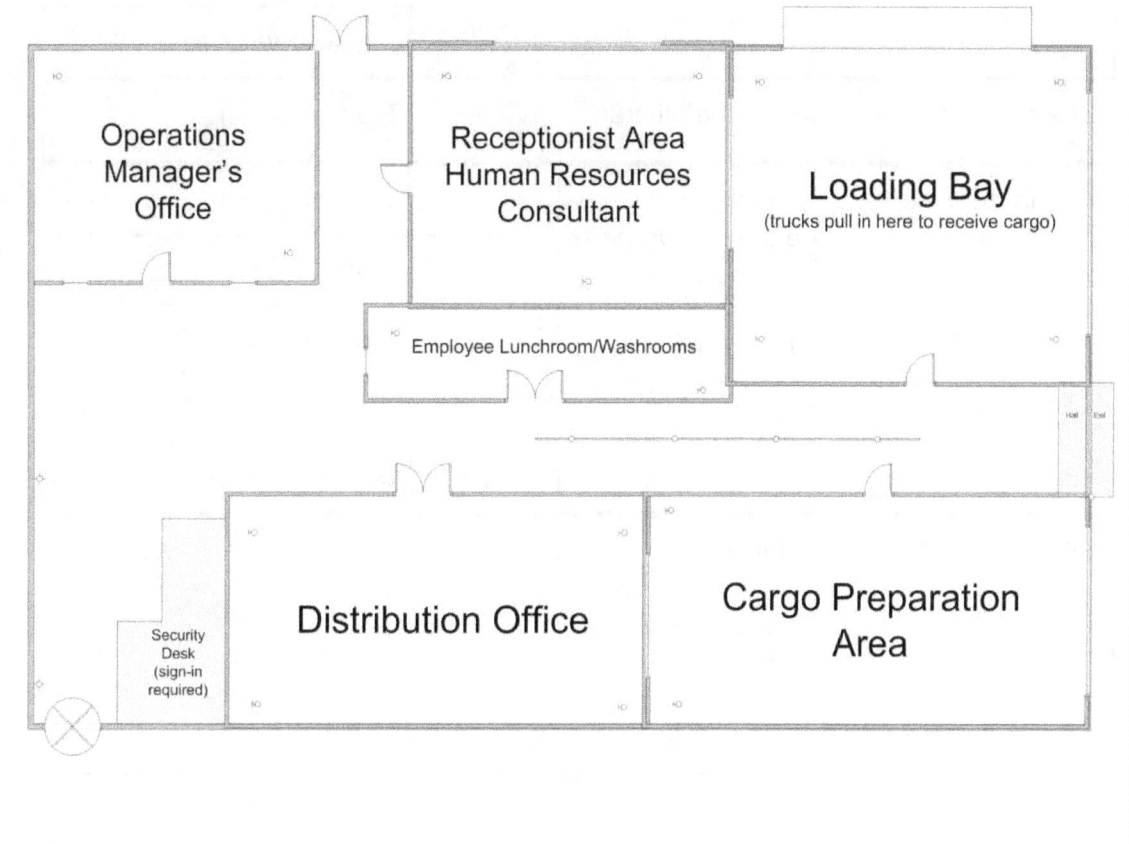

The staff and their hours are outlined below.

Staff Member	Responsibility	# of Staff	Hours Worked
Security guards	Patrol building and grounds every half hour. Monitor security desk and cameras.	2	7 am to 7 pm (Sun-Wed)
		2	7 am to 7 pm (Thu-Sat)
		2	7 pm to 7 am (Sun-Wed)
		2	7 pm to 7 am (Thu-Sat)
		1	Backup; varies
Operations manager	Oversee all staff.	1	8 am to 4 pm
Distribution clerks	Check invoices and prepare cargo. Transport cargo to loading bay.	2	7 am to 7 pm (Sun-Wed)
		1	7 am to 7 pm (Thu-Sat)
		2	7 pm to 7 am (Sun-Wed)
		1	7 pm to 7 am (Thu-Sat)
		1	Backup; varies
HR consultant	Manage all human resource issues, including personal counselling, hiring, firing.	1	8 am to 4 pm, although can be called in off-hours
Receptionist	Respond to incoming phone calls, e-mails, faxes. Prepare invoices and send to distribution clerks.	3	8 am to 4 pm
		2	4 pm to midnight
		1	Midnight to 6 a.m.
Warehouse Workers		4	8 am to 4 pm.

| | Let trucks into loading bay, place cargo onto trucks, and ensure paperwork is signed and cash received. | 4 | 4 pm to midnight. |
| | | 4 | Midnight to 6 a.m. |

Log of Safety Incidents

Incident	Date and Time	Action Taken
Truck driver backed into boxes in warehouse; boxes fell onto employee.	January 6, 2007 (Saturday) 7:19 p.m.	Employee taken to hospital; off work for 17 days.
Tape dispenser fell off top shelf of cargo preparation area; hit employee on head.	February 10, 2007, around 10 p.m.	None
Distribution clerk pulled back muscle moving box onto truck.	April 10, 2007 7:12 a.m.	Clerk off work permanently. Purchased forklift to assist with moving boxes.

Possible Hazards:

Hazards – What are they?

Living is about dealing with hazards. To understand any situation or task you are to perform, you need to understand what hazards are and how to deal with them.

A hazard is anything that can cause damage, injury or death. This potential may be small or big.

A hazard is therefore anything in this world or in its atmosphere that can be harmful, whether it is solid, liquid or gas.

Some hazards may be more dangerous than others.

No matter where you are, you are always surrounded by hazards. They are part of your everyday life.

Therefore a hazard is an actual object or substance, whether big or small, whether you can see, smell, touch, hear or taste it.

A situation can never be a hazard.

A situation can be hazardous or unsafe because hazards – objects or substances – that are present could cause damage, injury or death.

Hazards may be extremely big (like a mountain) or extremely small (like an ant or a virus).

- Sometimes you can only see it through a microscope.
- All hazards have mass (they have weight).
- They also have density (being solid, fluid or gas).
- They all have size (volume) and shape (square, round, sharp, etc.).
- Every hazard also has some form of energy.

So anything you make contact with may harm you.

Whether the situation in which the contact takes place is dangerous or not, depends on specific circumstances.

For example, an ant on a chair poses very little threat to most humans. However, an ant in your ear may be a different story.

Hazards are constantly interacting with one another. That means they come into contact with one another.

This happens during every moment of the day and the night.

Most interactions are planned in order to serve specific purposes, for example eating food (hazards) to supply energy, walking on pathways (hazards) to get somewhere, drilling a hole with something into something, the rays of the sun heating the earth, etc.

Types of hazards

There are three types of hazards:

- **A single hazard:** This is any single substance or physical element, e.g. iron and oxygen.
- **A compound hazard:** This is a mixture of hazards compiled in a single substance, e.g. a key, soap and the air you breathe.
- **A multiple hazard:** This is a combination of compound and / or single hazards in any proportion, e.g. a toolbox full of tools, or a motor vehicle.

Risk – The alerting factor

Everybody does not clearly understand what the term risk means.

> **Risk is the presence of uncertainty in a situation. All activities go with risk – some present more than others.**

Life is never without risk. However, risk does not mean that when an event will happen it will have negative results.

Risk means that harm to a person or damage to property may or is likely to occur.

Components of Risk

Risk has three components:

1. Frequency and duration of exposure

Exposure considers whether a task needs to be performed and, if so, how frequently will the exposure take place.

The following questions need to be answered:

- ➤ How many persons will perform the task?
- ➤ How long will it take to perform the task?
- ➤ How often or how many times will the task be performed in a given period or time?

2. Severity

Severity considers the possible consequences that are most likely to happen when a task is performed unsafe.

The consequences of the risk may be:

> ➢ Negligible – no or very little harm or damage,
> ➢ Marginal – minor injury, illness or damage,
> ➢ Critical – severe harm or damage,
> ➢ Catastrophic – permanent harm, death or huge losses.

3. Probability

Probability considers what the chances are that harm or damage may occur when one or more persons or workers will perform the task.

The key question is:

What is the possibility or how likely is it that harm or damage will occur when the task is done?

The probability or likelihood may be low, moderate or high. The level of risk associated with the task may therefore be low, moderate or high.

Interaction with hazard

- In order to interact safely, you need to identify the hazard (s) and assess the risk, i.e. likelihood of harm or damage, before you interact with a hazard.
- The type of force of the energy, which indicates the possible consequences during exposure, and the frequency of exposure spell out the risk.
- For this reason it is of great importance that you need to identify the hazard (s). The level of risk must alert you whether the interaction will be safe or not

Types of risk

There are various types of risk, namely pure risk and speculative risk.

Pure risk is risk that only result in loss, damage, disruption or injury. Pure risk can be divided into three categories:

- ❖ Inherent risk
- ❖ Add-on risk
- ❖ Unreasonable risk

Inherent Risk

Risk of harm or damage associated with a particular hazard, task or situation, is called inherent risk.
The risk in such a situation is created by the inherent characteristics of the hazard present and their interaction in that situation.

The level of risk, i.e. the possibility of loss as a result of the frequency and severity of exposure, may be low, moderate or high.

You can use countermeasures to reduce the frequency and severity of possible loss, but the countermeasures cannot change the level of the inherent risk. The level of risk is determined by the force of the energies as well as the frequency and duration of such energy.

Add-on Risk

Add-on risk is created by us humans. We do it through changing the original risk of an activity. This increases the chance of loss. The risk we may introduce may chance the original make-up of the object (hazard), task or activity.

Risk that we introduce into a situation and that is not part of the inherent risk of the hazards in such situation is called add-on risk.

Add-on risk is when we do not identify the hazards correctly, assess the risk improperly, misjudge our abilities to deal with the risk and perform the interaction process unsuccessfully.

Unreasonable risk – The worst

Unreasonable risk is a special type of inherent risk associated with a given hazard and the risk presented by the activity. When people directly interact with hazard that presents unreasonable risk, the chances of failure are almost certain.

An example is touching a live wire with an electrical current of 10 000 volts.

In the case of unreasonable risk, the following conditions exist:

- ❖ The probability of a failure is very likely,
- ❖ When failure occurs, loss will be significant,
- ❖ The person does not have the ability to interact with the hazard directly,
- ❖ Countermeasures can be introduced to reduce the unreasonable risk to an acceptable level.

Housekeeping / Order

Housekeeping is second nature to a good skill but, looking at housekeeping practices throughout industry, one questions the skills of our supervisors and workers.

Definition of order: A place is in order when there are no unnecessary things about, and when all necessary things are in their proper places.

Definition of housekeeping: Housekeeping is a place for everything and everything in its place.

Personal Protective Equipment (PPE) Legal References

- Take reasonable care of his / her own health and safety,
- Co-operate with the employer to ensure that the requirements, as set out in the OHS Act and the regulations are fulfilled,
- The employer may not deduct the cost of PPE issued to any employee from the employee's wage.

This does not mean that an employee may abuse the PPE without any worry. This could be committing an offence in terms of Section 15 and can result in the employee having to pay.

Body parts to be protected and common types of PPE

Body Part	PPE
Head	Hard hats and hair nets
Eyes	Safety goggles / glasses (various types)
Ears	Ear muffs and plugs
Arms	Long gloves / overalls
Hands	Gloves
Body	Overalls and Aprons
Legs	Overalls
Feet	Safety Shoes / boots
Lungs	Dust masks / respirators
Skin	Barrier cream / Overalls
Kidneys	Kidney belts
	Safety Harnesses

Requirements for PPE:

- SABS standards
- OHS Act standards
- SAPEMA standards
- BS – DIN – ANSI – etc.

PPE must;

- Fit comfortably
- Give you adequate protection
- Be readily available

How to know which PPE to be used

- HIRA studies should be conducted,
- The employee should be taught in his workplace which PPE is required for his job and the hazard it is meant to protect him against,
- His supervisor should ensure that he is issued with the correct type of PPE,
- He should be trained in the correct use and the limitation of PPE,
- The employee must use his direction and request PPE if, in his opinion, it is necessary to protect him against a possible hazards,
- The employee must wear, and look after, his PPE in the same way he looks after himself.

Supervisor's Responsibility

- Conduct hazard identification and risk assessment (HIRA) studies,
- Enforce the wear of PPE,
- Set the example,
- Involve is people in decision making; empower them,
- Conduct behavioural interviews.

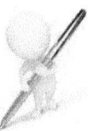

Activity 9: Acme Widget Company

Earlier we looked at the Acme Widget Company and identified some possible safety hazards. Look back at that list and identify some ways of resolving those hazards.

Hazard	Engineering Controls	Work Practices	PPE

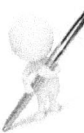

Activity 10: HEALTH AND SAFETY

1. Identify any other health and safety issues in your premises.
2. Customize the Health and Safety Checklist provided for your business.
3. Draw up an action plan of steps you need to implement with regards to health and safety issues in your business.

Action	By Who?	By When?

1. Devise a list of health and safety rules / policy. Communicate this to your staff.

Writing a Safety Plan

Now that you have a safety committee, you can write a safety plan. Safety Plan must consist of the following:

- Written policy,
- Guidelines,
- Description of the organisation,
- Arrangements of carrying out and reviewing the policy
- Displayed,
- Signed.

Implementing the Plan

Now that the safety plan has been written, it's time to implement it. Where do you start?

- Go over the plan with all employees.
- Put the plan in place immediately.
- If there are many, many changes to be made, these may have to be implemented slowly. Start with the biggest hazards.
- Set a good example by modeling safety yourself.

Incident Management

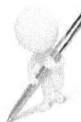

Activity 11: Case Study

No matter how well your safety culture is implemented and accepted, there will still be incidents. Read this case study and think of how you would respond if you were in the factory at the time of the incident.

Case Study

Inside a meat packing plant, twenty workers are all performing various tasks involving heavy machinery. Suddenly, a scream echoes through the factory. George, the foreman, has gotten his arm caught in one of the meat packing machines. Panic erupts: one worker turns to stare and gets caught in the conveyor belt; another worker trips and falls as he tries to run from the scene; yet another worker falls into the vat that they have been cleaning out. No one has called for help and the scene is in complete chaos.

What would you do if you were working in the factory?

Principles of Accident Prevention

Accident prevention is the main objective of:

- Occupational Health and Safety Act.
- Mine Health and Safety Act.
- Explosives Act.

What is an Incident?

An incident is an undesired event that could (or does) downgrade the efficiency or the business operation.

What is an Accident?

An accident is an undesired event mainly caused by unsafe behaviour and / or unsafe physical conditions that result in physical harm to a person or in damage to property.

Usually it is the result of contact with a source of energy, i.e. kinetic, electrical, thermal, etc., above the threshold limit of the human body or structure.

COID Act defines an accident as arising out of and in the course of a person's employment resulting in a personal injury. These two definitions are contradictory.

What is a near-miss incident?

These incidents are frequently referred to as near-miss accidents and in most cases the use of terms is quite accurate.

Except for the severity there is actually no difference between an incident, an accident or a near-miss accident. In all three cases the immediate causes (unsafe behaviour and / or unsafe conditions), as well as the root causes (personal and job-related factors), were present.

Causes and effects of downgrading incidents

To understand the sequences of events that can lead to an undesired loss, it is essential that we understand what it is we are trying to prevent or control.

It could be problems arising from:

- Safety
- Health
- Environment
- Fire
- Production
- Security

Circumstances that lead to loss

The four major elements or subsystems in the business operation – people, equipment, material and environment – individual, or in combination, provide the source of causes that contribute to downgrading incidents.

Lack of Control – Management

- Inadequate programme,
- Inadequate programme standards,
- Failure to comply with standards,
- Inform management on OHS Act, COID Act and other related statutes.

The word control here refers to any of the four functions of any professional manager:

- Planning
- Leading
- Organising
- Controlling

If these functions are specifically related to an OH&S programme, the programme will include:

- Making inspections,
- Conducting group meetings,
- Indoctrinating new employees,
- Doing investigations,
- Doing a job analysis,
- Reviewing rules and procedures,
- Giving proper job instruction.

Reasons for Safety

- Legal requirement,
- Company requirement,
- Good practice requirement,
- Moral obligation,
- Financial consideration.

Types of Losses

- People losses,
- Asset losses,
- Liability losses,
- Net income losses.

Human Behaviour during a fire

Compliance with fire safety requirement of building regulations, Occupational Health and Safety Act, standards and codes would no doubt reduce the fire risk in a building and provide adequate means of safe evacuation. The success of these measures, however, depends to the great extent on the behaviour of building occupancy at the time of the fire. Buildings contain a variety of people, some who will be able to escape in most circumstances, others who would have extreme difficulty, and those who will not attempt to escape, among which some will take risk of fighting the fire. These facets of behaviour are influenced by psychological, physiological, and circumstantial factors and previous involvement in fire incidents. They can also be influenced by the severity of the threat posed by the fire, the building design and the fire protection devices installed.

Main conclusion:

1. The behaviour of an individual can be modified according to the role in which the individual sees himself or herself and whether that role is part of a strong hierarchy: in office blocks, managers behave differently from guests; in hospital, staff continue duties to patients. Confusion would result in the fire intelligence and action flow conflicted with normal hierarchy.
2. Building occupants do not use escape routes that are unfamiliar to them. This implies that purpose-build fire escapes might be less than wholly effective, particularly to those unfamiliar with the building.
3. Fire extinguishers are rarely used and are not effective. Without training, many have difficulty in using extinguishers.
4. The earliest cues to fire are generally strange noises like breaking glass and extra activity by others, rather than flame or smoke.
5. Early behaviour is characterized by uncertainty, misinterpretation, and indecisiveness and seeking additional information for confirmation – the "gathering phase". Such delay can be dangerous, as actions taken at the early stages of a fire have the most decisive effect on the eventual outcome.
6. The response to fire alarm bells and sounders tend to be less than optimum. There is usually scepticism as to whether the noise indicated a fire alarm and if so, is the alarm merely a system test or drill?
7. In the stress of fire, people can often act inappropriate and panic or behave irrationally. Such behaviour, to a large extend, is due to the fact the information initially available to people regarding possible existence of a fire and its size and location is often ambiguous or inadequate.

Planning

A properly planned and regularly practiced procedure is necessary for all buildings, so that occupants will know how to make an efficient and orderly escape during an emergency. Evacuation can only be successfully undertaken if there are well-constructed marked exits in the building, with the aid of well-trained emergency marshals.

Objectives

- Two and a half minutes is the average time for anyone to reach a place of safety. This time may vary from building to building depending in the size, number and type of occupants.
- No one should go towards a fire to escape. An alternative route must always be available.
- Everyone should be able to escape by his or her own unaided efforts. Special attention will have to be given to aged, ill or non-ambient occupants. Many companies have day care centres for their employees' children and here special attention will have to be given.
- Escape routes should lead directly to a place of safety.
- A place of safety in an area where people can disperse – it may be outside, in other compartments, a protected staircase or lobby.
- To reveal weaknesses in the plans and procedures before emergencies occur.
- To identify deficiencies in resources (both in manpower and equipment).
- To improve the level of co-ordination among various response personnel, departments and agencies.
- To regain public recognition and confidence in the ability to manage emergency situations.
- To improve the proficiency and confidence of emergency response personnel.
- To clarify each individual's role and areas of responsibility.
- To enhance overall emergency response capabilities.

Considerations

In planning evacuation procedures, the following must be considered:

1. The possible behaviour of a fire with special regard to the spread of smoke.
2. The type of risk and number occupants. People may either be sleeping, be unfamiliar with the building or be very young or aged.
3. The building contents could facilitate rapid fire spread.
4. The exit widths must accommodate the occupants to enable them to evacuate within two and a half minutes.
5. Emergency lifting and generators in the case of total or partial power failure.
6. Warning signs with the following instruction "DO NOT USE THE LIFT IN CASE OF FIRE" to be posted at each lift door on every floor.
7. Assembly points and toll call registers.

Additional considerations

1. An alarm system is essential to initiate evacuation procedures.
2. Moving machinery, fuel and gas lines and electrical should be shut down, or important documents should be put into fire safe cabinets by a designated person (s) prior to evacuation.
3. Offices must be numbered, this will enable the person reporting the fire or emergency to pinpoint its exact location accurately. It will enable the emergency personnel to move directly to the fire or emergency area.
4. High risk areas should be clearly identified, this will enable the emergency personnel to make clear and decisive decisions on the emergency procedure that has to be followed. If necessary, additional training must be provided to handle such an area safely.

5. First aid training and equipment for marshals, should medical assistance be required during evacuation.

Procedures

The evacuation plan must be circulated to occupants and management, details must be displayed on each section floor and / or within each section. This evacuation plan must be a floor plan stating where the occupancy is and clearly showing he escape routes and the alternative escape route to be used.

Emergency procedure instructions and telephone numbers must be posted by each telephone. It is necessary to appoint a Chief Fire Marshal to direct operations (usually from a control centre). Fire marshals on each floor / department floor can supervise evacuations, initially attack the fire and assist the Chief Fire Marshal.

Evacuation Procedures

If a multi-storey is to be completely evacuated, the following events should be followed as closely as possible.

When a fire breaks out, people in the emergency centre – in this case the reception area on the ground floor – are notified. They must obtain the following information:

1. The location and nature of the fire.
2. Whether there are any injuries or medical emergencies.

THEY WILL THEN:

1. Inform the Fire Brigade with the following information:
   - Who is calling (name, surname and telephone number)
   - Where the fire is:
     - ❖ Name of the business and or building name and number of the building.
     - ❖ Street name
     - ❖ Nearest Cross street.
     - ❖ Suburb.
     - ❖ What is the nature of the fire?
     - ❖ Medical Emergencies
2. Initiate the evacuation alarm.
3. Recall all lifts to the ground floor and lock them.
4. Contact the Chief Fire Marshal.

THE CHIEF FIRE MARSHAL WILL THEN:

1. Take charge of the emergency centre.
2. Co-ordinate the evacuation and activities of fire teams and control building services such as lifts, emergency generators, emergency lighting and central air conditioner plants.
3. Liaise with the Fire Department.

ON THE FIRE FLOOR, THE MARSHALS WILL:

1. Begin evacuating employees
   Employees evacuating will ensure the following:
   - Immediately on hearing the evacuation alarm, lock away important documents in fire safe cabinets.
   - Collect personal belongings such as car keys, handbags and brief cases.
   - Switch off electrical equipment such as air conditioners and computers.
   - Close all open windows in an office.
   - Check emergency plan as reminder of escape routes and alternative escape routes.
   - Upon leaving office, close the door, DO NOT LOCK.
   - If a marshal is not in sight, move to the most safest and direct escape route. REMEMBER: DO NOT RUN, WALK BRISKLY AND TRY TO MOVE IN GROUPS OF TWO OR MORE IN A SINGLE FILE. ALWAYS LISTEN TO THE EVACUATION MARSHAL.
   - FOR NO REASON RETURN TO THE OFFICE ONCE YOU HAVE STARTED TO EVACUATE.
   - When you leave the building, report to the assembly point immediately for roll call. Once the emergency is over, personnel will be dismissed to return to their workstations or to go home. This will only happen when the "all clear" has been given by the Fire Department, Chief Fire Marshal or management, whichever is applicable.

2. Attack the fire if expedient to do so – REMEMBER: IF IN DOUBT, DO NOT ATTEMPT TO FIGHT THE FIRE, and EVACUATE THE BUILDING.

THE DUTIES OF THE FIRE MARSHAL DURING AN EMERGENCY:

- Muster occupants and guide them to the correct exits.
- Prevent people from returning for personal belongings.
- Prevent people from using lifts.
- Control congestion in stairways.
- Search floor areas, toilets and landings between floors.
- Close doors, particularly staircase doors.
- Report to Chief Fire Marshal that the floor is clean.
- Guide occupants to assembly area.
- Take roll call.

ACTIONS WHEN BUILDING BECOMES SMOKE LOGGED

- If possible, tie a damp handkerchief around your nose and mouth. This action will filter the air of toxic gasses, and cool down the air breathed in.
- Go on your hands and knees and crawl as close as possible to the wall. If possible, stay away from the centre of the floor as it may have been weakened due to the fire and could possibly collapse.
- If your vision becomes impaired due to smoke, use the left of right hand for evacuation.
- Whilst crawling, close your hands with your thumbs on the outside of your fists.
- Whilst evacuating you encounter a closed door, do not open the door directly. Feel whether the door is hot by using the back of your hand.

- When encountering stairs descent by crawling down backwards, keeping as close as possible to the side of the wall.
- REMEMBER: STAY CLOSE TO THE FLOOR. THAT IS WHERE THE AIR WILL BE THE LEAST TOXIC. DO NOT PANIC.

ACTIONS WHEN TRAPPED IN A BURNING BUILDING

- If you become trapped in a burning building, enter a office which is not burning, close the door and try and seal the door by using available material i.e. jackets, rugs or carpets.
- Try to attract the attention of people on the outside of the building.
- If you cannot attract attention, lay done in the corner of the office, preferably the left hand corner closest to the door when entering. Force yourself to calm down and breathe regularly.
- Use a hard instrument (if possible, metal) and tap against the floor, wall or piping that might run through the office to attract attention. Use the international SOS signal. Three rapid taps, three slow taps, three rapid taps.
- If you are not higher than the first storey of a building, the following steps can be taken to escape:
  - ❖ Tie curtains, belts and thick electrical cords together, tie these to a secure point close to the window, i.e. heavy piece of furniture.
  - ❖ Lower yourself hand over hand until you reach the ground or as far as possible, then drop the rest of the distance.

Bombs:
- Time permitting, assemble the ECPC and place wardens on standby;
- Notify the SAPS;
- Evaluate the credibility of the bomb threat on the basis of all available information [i.e. complete Bomb threat checklist, political situation, Police warning, etc.]
- Order a search of work stations by people employed at those places work stations [time permitting] if the location of the bomb is known or hinted at, search that area first;
- If a bomb or suspicious article is found or if the bomb threat is regarded as credible and time does not permit search- **EVACUATE!!**

In the event of an explosion, activate fire and casualty situation plans.

Safety Signs

Colour Coding: Plant and Pipelines

Painting different areas and pipes in different colours makes it easy for everyone to identify the purpose or contents immediately. It is then easy to know if the pipe contains material that is hazardous or not. This is especially important for maintenance staff and contractors.

Each company should have colour coding boards which show what each colour means. These should be used at induction training and displayed in appropriate departments and at several points throughout the plant.

Notices and Signs

Colour coding and symbolic signs have similar purposes. The use of symbolic safety signs makes it easy for everyone to understand the information instantly.

Signs are made up of three different parts:

- ❖ The shape
- ❖ The colour (s)
- ❖ The pictogram (picture)

GEOMETRIC SHAPES:

	Warning	Yellow
	Prohibitory	Red
	Mandatory	Blue
	Information (General)	Green
	Information (Fire Equipment)	White

COLOURS

RED:

- Danger.
- Fire Protection Equipment.
- Stop Buttons and controls.

YELLOW:

- Places where care must be taken,
- Warning of radio-active substances.

BLUE:

- Mandatory signs – i.e. information about PPE requirements.

GREEN:

- Green and white is for general information.

WHITE:

- Location.

BLACK:

- Hazard / death.

ORANGE:

- Electrical Equipment.

EXAMPLES OF INFORMATION, FIRE FIGHTING SIGNAGE

For Fire Equipment / Emergency Equipment

Shape: Square
Colour: White with red border line
Pictogram: Red

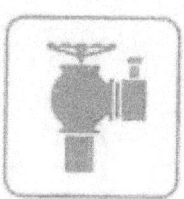 Fire Hydrant

 Location of Fire Blanket

 Fire Hose

 Location of fire-fighting equipment

 Fire Extinguisher

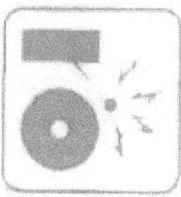 Fire Alarm

 Fire Marshal

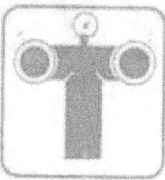 Fire Pump Connection

 Fire Telephone

 Sprinkler Stop Valve

EXAMPLES OF WARNING SIGNAGES

Yellow and black signs tell you to be careful.

It is warning you!

Shape: Triangular
Colour: Black Border, yellow centre
Pictogram: Black

 Warning Biological Hazard

 Warning of hazard of cold burns

 Warning of corrosive hazard

 Warning of Carbon dioxide hazard

 General Warning

 Beware of dogs

 Warning of explosion hazard

 Warning of Fire Hazard

 Beware of Forklifts
high

 Warning of hazard of exposed live
voltage equipment

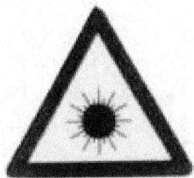 Warning of Laser hazard

 Warning of suspended loads hazard

 Warning of moving machinery moving

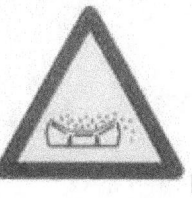 Beware of material falling from conveyor belt

 Warning of methane hazard substances

 Warning of poisonous

 Warning of ionizing radiation

 Warning of fragile roof

 General Warning of electrical shock

 Warning of hazard of slippery walking surface

 Warning of hazard of slippery steps

 Warning of workers overhead

 Warning of asbestos hazard

EXAMPLES OF MANDATORY SIGNAGE

They tell you what protective equipment you need to wear in that area.

It is compulsory!
Shape: Circular (disc)
Colour: Blue
Pictogram: White

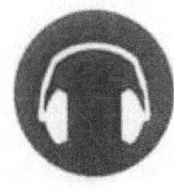 Hearing Protection shall be worn liquids

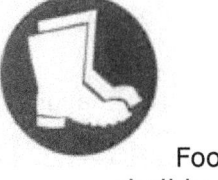 Foot and leg protection against shall be worn

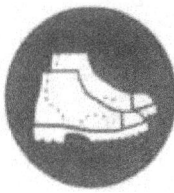 Foot protection against crushing shall be worn

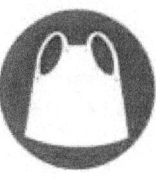 Apron shall be worn

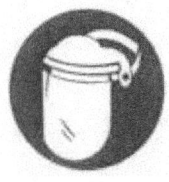 Face protection shall be worn

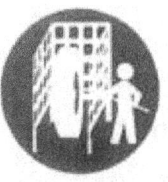 Use safety cage

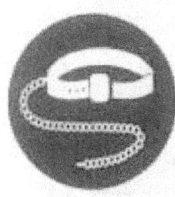 Safety harnesses / lifeline shall be worn

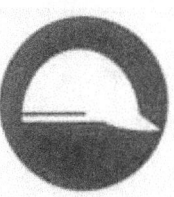 Head protection shall be worn

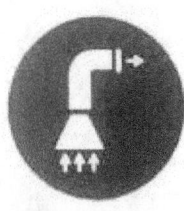 Air extraction shall be used worn

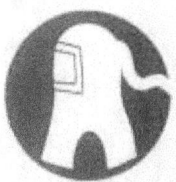 Air-supplied hood shall be worn

 Hand protection shall be worn

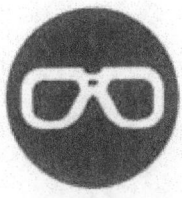 Eye protection shall be worn

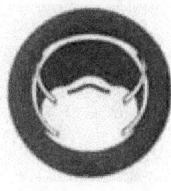 Dust mask shall be worn

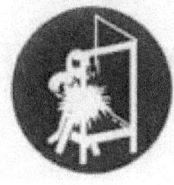 screening to be used

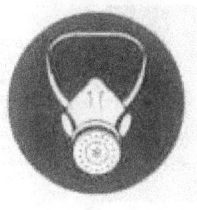 Respirator protection shall be worn

EXAMPLES OF INFORMATION, GENERAL SIGNAGE

These are for information or direction.

Green and white signs shows us where service areas are.

Shape:	Square
Colour:	Green
Pictogram:	White

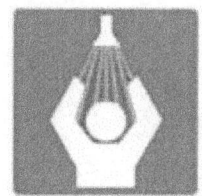 Safety Shower

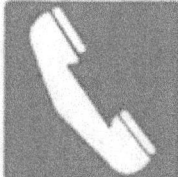 Telephone

 Traveling way

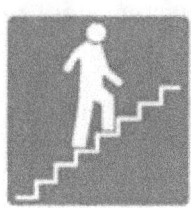 Stairs going up

 Waiting place   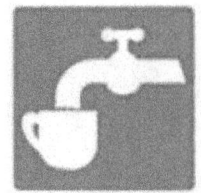 Drinking water

EXAMPLES OF PROHIBITION SIGNAGE

They say Danger!

Stop and Think!

Shape: Circular (annular / disc)
Colour: White with red border line and oblique diametric line
Pictogram: Black

 Thoroughfare for pedestrians prohibited    Hand tramming prohibited

 Fire and open flames prohibited    No entry for heavy
vehicles

 Water as extinguisher agent prohibited   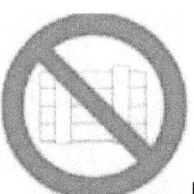 Do not obstruct

 Carrying of long material prohibited    Smoking prohibited

Demarcation

Demarcation means different areas are marked off. Each area is for different materials or jobs. In the factory, workshop or plant, lines are painted on the floor. These lines show where it is safe to walk. Where the forklifts can drive. Lines also show where to load materials and pallets. Where emergency equipment is.

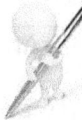

Activity 12:

12.1 What is the purpose of safety signs?
12.2 What steps should you take to prepare for the possibility of fires?
12.3 Describe the importance of fire exits.
12.4 Draw up a reference sheet for all the emergency signs and list their meanings.

Injury and Accident Reporting

Accidents are the results of hazardous acts or hazardous conditions – most often a combination of both.

Objective:

The Employer must have an effective Accident / Incident Investigation programme, which methodically examines all undesired events that have or could have resulted in physical harm to employees, damage to property, and loss to process or pollution to the environment.

Aims of these investigations:

The aims of these investigations are to:

1. Establish facts and circumstances related to the event.
2. Determine the root and basic cause and,
3. Develop remedial actions to prevent further risks,
4. Improve a supervisor's management approach,
5. Comply with policies and statutory requirements,
6. Maintain employee awareness of the importance of safe, healthy work habits,
7. Prevent recurrence.

DEFINITIONS

Accident:	An unexpected, unplanned occurrence that results in injury or harm to persons, property or the environment.
Causes:	Any unsafe act or condition that contribute to an accident or "near-miss".
Change analysis:	A process used to determine the cause of an accident by comparing the way a job was actually performed with the way it should have been performed.
Incident:	The term is often used to refer to both accident and incidents. An unexpected, unplanned occurrence that results in injury or harm to persons, property or the environment.
Job Hazard Analyses (JHA):	A method in which job steps are identified, hazards are determined, and solutions are recommended to eliminate or control those hazards.
Near-Miss Accident:	An unexpected, unplanned occurrence that does not cause injury or loss, but which has the potential for doing so.
Occupational Disease:	A disease caused by exposure to environmental; factors associated with employment. Work related disability includes such ailments as silicosis, pneumoconiosis and loss of hearing. Even though there is no traumatic injury in such disabilities, if they are work related they are considered on duty injuries.
Physical Evidence:	The condition and / or position of equipment and materials at the scene of an accident that can provide information to deduce what actually happened.
SOP's:	Standard Oprating Procedures – an established method of performing a specific job or task in the most effective and safe way.

Root Causes – Origins

Existence of personal and job factors.
Root (Basic) causes are frequently classified into two groups:

PERSONAL FACTORS	JOB FACTORS
Lack of knowledge or skill.	Inadequate design.
Improper motivations.	Inadequate work standards.
Physical or mental problems.	Inadequate purchasing.
	Normal wear and tear.
	Abnormal usage.

Root (Basic) causes are the origin of unsafe acts and conditions, however this is not the beginning of the "cause and effect" sequence. The sequence begins with the lack of control, which will present itself in one of the following:

Inadequate programme:	the SHE programme may be inadequate because of too few programme activities.
Inadequate programme standards:	a common cause of standards failing is that they are not specific enough.
Inadequate compliance with standards:	a common reason for lack of control.

A thorough investigation should expose failures in the:

- SHE programme
- Standards
- Compliance with the respective standard and by addressing the problem at this level one will ensure that problems do not recur.

Experience has shown that causes of accidents are often multiple i.e. a single event is not the only cause and that the opportunity for control is also multiple.

Immediate Causes – Symptoms

Existence of substandard practices and conditions occurrence of errors:

UNSAFE PRACTICES	UNSAFE CONDITIONS
Operating without authority.	Inadequate guards.
Failure to warn or secure.	Defective tools.
Using defective equipment.	Congestion.
Failure to wear PPE.	Bad housekeeping.
Improper lifting.	Excessive noise.
Horseplay.	Inadequate lighting.
Taking drugs.	Hazardous atmosphere.
Not using safety devices.	Radiation exposure.

Incident - Contact

An undesired event that could or does make contact with a source of energy above the threshold limit of body or structure.

Common types of accidents:

- Struck against,
- Struck by,
- Fall to below,
- Fall to same level,
- Caught in,
- Caught on,
- Caught between,
- Contact with source of energy,
- Overexertion (overload).

People and Property – Loss

Physical Harm	Property Harm
Minor	Minor
Serious	Serious
Reportable	Major
Compensatable	Catastrophic
Disabling	
Fatal	
Catastrophic	

Losses involved with all areas of the business activity could be considered as above for physical harm and property damage, as well as humane effects and economic aspects.

Investigate near misses

Today's close call could be tomorrow's serious accident. It is important to investigate close calls. A near miss should be considered an accident that didn't happen. Its causes have to be identified and eliminated, otherwise the next near miss could be the next serious accident.

Accident investigation is part of almost every SHE programme. Yet, the purpose for doing investigations is often poorly understood. As a result it can degenerate into a finger-pointing, blame-fixing and fault-finding exercise, which neither determines the real reason for what happened nor arrives at any effective solution to the problem involved.

An effective investigation can:

- Describe what happened,
- Determine the root causes,
- Decide the risks,
- Develop control,
- Define trends,
- Demonstrate concern.

Even when the purpose is properly defined, investigations are often executed poorly. Perhaps the greatest reason for this is, not understanding the many real values to be gained.

What should be investigated?

Look at the objectives of the OHS Act.

OHS Act:

To provide for the health and safety of persons at work and for the health and safety of persons in connection with the use of plant and machinery.

In terms of the three statutes, the following should be investigated:

- Fatal injuries
- Disabling injuries
- Occupational Injuries
- Reportable injuries
- Minor injuries
- Property damage
- Machinery incidents etc.

All incidents / accidents and near misses should be investigated. All immediate and basic causes are present in the above examples, the only difference being the severity.

Who should be investigated?

As with any type of problem solving, the person with the most interest in the mishap is the obvious first choice. A person with a vital interest finds solutions that work.

Another important consideration in the choice of the investigator is that he must be able to stay objective.

The Line Supervisors

Supervisors are busy people with lots to do. Is it reasonable to involve them in investigations? Absolutely!

Most of their time is spent on problem solving. Investigating incidents and accidents is not only their responsibility, it is their right.

- Supervisors have personal interest,
- They know the people and conditions,
- They know best how and where to get the necessary information,
- They benefit from investigating,
- It increases production,
- It shows that supervisors have control.

Middle Managers

Sometimes investigations require participation by middle and high-level managers (statutory appointees.

Cases where middle managers participate in investigations:

- Major loss or potential incidents,
- Where circumstances cross into other supervisors' areas,
- The remedial actions have a broad scope of significant costs.

Other persons

The following persons should be or could be involved:

- SHE practitioner,
- Health and safety representatives,
- Competent person (machinery),
- Occupational health nurse,
- Witnesses,
- Injured,
- Social worker / HR personnel.

Sequence

A guide to follow for incident reporting, recording, investigation, analysis and costing:

- Accident / incident notification,
- Care and treatment of injured,
- Managing the accident scene,
- Identifying witnesses,
- Preliminary investigation,
- Reporting to authorities, if necessary,
- Loss announcement,
- Formal company investigation.
- Supervisors can investigate only the incidents / accidents they know about.
- Notification procedures should be posted conspicuously in the work areas and should include names and contact numbers of personnel who may need to be contacted.
- Five minute safety talks / induction training!!

CAUSATION MODEL

ACCIDENT

LACK OF CONTROL

SYMPTOMS

UNSAFE ACT

UNSAFE CONDITIONS

Basic causes explain why unsafe acts and conditions occur

BASIC CAUSE

INCIDENT CONTACT

BASIC CAUSES

BASIC CAUSES

LOSS CAUSATION MODEL

LACK OF CONTROL	BASIC CAUSES	IMMEDIATE CAUSES	INCIDENT	LOSS
• Inadequate Systems • System Standards • Compliance	• Personal Factors • Job Factors	• Sub Standards and Conditions	• Contact with energy • Substance • Process or people	• Inadequate Systems • System standards • Compliance

PRE-CONTACT PHASE	CONTACT PHASE	POST CONTACT PHASE
• Vulnerability profiling. • Job hazard analysis, SOP's, Job Observations. • Planned Inspections. • Contractor Safety. • Job planning, Hazard Identification and Investigation.	Accident / Incident	Emergency Crisis Management

Care and treatment of injured

In most instances, the care and treatment of the injured will come first.

When injuries are encountered at the accident scene, the supervisor should make sure that proper emergency help has been summoned and the victim receives the necessary first aid.

Training employees as first responders, or certification in emergency care and CPR, could make the difference between life and death at an accident scene.

Managing the accident scene

Without proper management, an accident scene can be confusing and chaotic place, particular when injuries are involved.

The supervisor responsible for the area should take charge of the site and direct any response activities.
- Care and treatment of injured,
- Eliminating or control of remaining hazards.

When hazardous substances at the scene present an immediate threat to the health and safety of anyone, eliminating or controlling the hazard should come first.

The site where the accident occurred must not be disturbed and the areas should be demarcated with chevron tape. Bystanders should be controlled to protect people and preserve evidence.

Witnesses

- Identify witnesses who can provide input in the investigation.
- Conditions at the scene can often provide valuable clues as to what occurred and why.
- Take photos – a camera is one of the investigators most versatile and useful tools.

General uses of photographs:

- Orientation to the scene of the accident.
- Record of detail of injury and damage.
- Details of marks, spills, instructional aids, signs, etc.
- Locations of parts, or other evidence, overlooked during early stages of investigation.

Identification of elements at the scene of the accident

Much evidence is lost to the investigation because it is removed or altered at the accident site before any notice of it is taken or any record is made.

The following elements should be noted during the initial identification of evidence:

- People
- Equipment
- Material
- Environment

People involved:	Injured, principals and witnesses.
Equipment involved:	In use, standby and secured, and PPE.
Material involved:	In use, ready for use and stored in the area.
Environmental factors:	Weather, lighting, heat, noise, fumes, dust, etc.

Gathering of information

Facts concerning an accident must be reported before an investigation can be completed. The information that will be required includes:

- The nature of any injuries.
- Property damage, or environmental harm that may have resulted.
- Where the accident happened?
- When it happened?
- Who was involved?

Witness Interviews and Statements

During the interview, the investigator should introduce "control" questions to insure accuracy of statistical data as well as permit subsequent evaluation of the reliability of information supplied by the witness. The control questions should include:

- Time and location of the accident.
- Environment: weather, lighting, temperature, noise, distracters, and concealments. Include pre-contact, contact and post-contact time periods by specific questions.
- Positions of people, equipment material and their relationships to pre-contact, contact and post-contact events. Include the position of the witness being interviewed.
- Other witnesses, know as well as those unidentified by name, and their positions.
- If anything was moved, repositioned, turned off or on, or taken from the scene, during pre-contact and post-contact phases.
- Observations of the response of emergency teams and supervisory personnel and their actions at the scene.
- What attracted the witness' attention to the accident?
- What the witness would do to prevent getting involved in a similar accident under similar circumstances.

The time, location, environment, position and witnesses are factual data that are needed to make a word picture of the accident for the report. These items are also valuable in analyzing the credibility of the witness as an observer.

Physical Evidence

The careful examination of the condition of equipment, materials and the environment at an accident scene can be critical to determine the cause of an accident. This physical evidence will often provide information about an accident that witnesses cannot.

Paper Evidence

Paper lead to a thorough examination of the policies, standards and specifications that moulded the environment, that forged the attitudes and actions of people involved in the accident. They show irrefutable evidence that generally does not come out in verbal testimony. Paper evidence, for clarity of discussion, is defined to encompass those documents, formal and informal, which contain information about the people, equipment, material and environment as related to the accident.

Often there are a wide variety of written records that can be reviewed. It is appropriate to examine the ones that can ask specific questions that develop during the analysis phase of the investigation. The three most common types of existing records are:

- **Employee records:** such as employment and health records, licenses, certificates and training records.
- **Equipment records:** including maintenance logs, service reports, operating manuals and manufacturer's instructions and safety specifications and requirements.
- **Job or task records:** standard operating procedures and job hazard analysis, for example; previous accident investigation reports / Incident Recall – investigations into similar accidents or near-misses may provide clues about the causes of the accident under investigation. While it is important to obtain witness accounts and examine the scene as soon as possible, reviewing written records and documents can usually wait until operations have been returned to normal.

Report to authorities

Reporting to authorities should be done timeously on prescribed forms:

1. Report to Inspector (OHS Act).
2. Report to Commissioner (COID Act).
3. SAPS (Unnatural Death Act).

Conducting an Accident Investigation

An accident investigation should begin as soon as possible after an accident has occurred. There are at least three reasons why this is important;

- Operations are disrupted; The more serious an accident is, the more time and effort it takes to bring work back to normal. The sooner an accident investigation begins, the sooner the operation can resume.
- Memories fade: As time passes, what a person remembers can change. Interviewing witnesses as soon as possible after the accident helps assure a more accurate account of what happened.
- Employees are at risk: If an accident happened once, there is a good chance that it can happen again unless the causes are identified and corrected, The sooner an investigation can determine the causes of an accident, the sooner corrective actions can be taken to prevent a recurrence.

Corrective Actions and Writing the Report

Temporary Actions: As they respond to and investigate incidents, supervisors should keep in mind the question, "What can I do right now to prevent this accident from happening again?" Most temporary actions correct only the symptoms – the substandard actions and conditions. There is nothing wrong with that. It's good place to start and it needs to be done. The worn out tools needs to be replaced, the cluttered floor needs to be cleaned up.

.

Permanent Actions: Permanent actions are required to solve the problem effectively and to ensure that the personal factors and the job factors are remedied in terms of the basic causes. Because time, materials and cost estimations are needed the action normally starts with the line management.

A risk assessment, looking at the degree of risk involved, will determine the combination of its severity and its likelihood of recurrence and will assist the investigator in marking practical recommendations.

The potential severity of an accident or incident is not determined by just what happened, It is determined by what the consequences are likely to be if it happened again. Because an undesirable event that produced only minor loss has the realistic potential to or a fatality, as well as significant property damage, it has high potential severity. Probability of recurrence is determined by asking how likely the accident or incident is to occur again if no corrective action is taken.

Thus, each recommendation should be guided by the risk involved in the situation and how much the recommendation action reduces it. Accidents and incidents, which have a high severity potential and high likelihood of happening again, will receive more extensive correction than those with low severity potential and low likelihood of ever occurring again. Corrective actions that significantly reduce one or both of these factors, i.e., makes it less likely to recur or reduce the severity if it does recur, are of greater value than corrective actions, which have small impact on these factors. Risk evaluation is a critical tool in making decisions and setting priorities.

Writing the report:

The report puts the investigation all together in a brief summary. It communicates the critical facts to the employees who have to act on them. It makes a record, which has many uses in the Risk Control programme. Also, it gives feedback to help appraise supervisor's performance in problem solving.

Writing a good report:

Use words that are common, short and specific. Follow this guide:

1. **Identify information:** Fill in all spaces in your report.
2. **Evaluation:** What was the real potential for loss (not just what happened)? If no corrective action is taken, how often can it be expected to occur?
3. **Description:** Tell what you have decided actually happened, what actions led up to the incident, the contact and what was done post contact to reduce the loss?

4. **Cause analysis:** List the symptoms (the substandard actions and conditions) and the basic causes (the job factors and personal factors). Give a few words explaining each cause. In listing basic causes, list first those that made the greatest contribution to the accident.

5. **Action plan:** Write first a short sentence or a few words stating what was done right away. Then write your recommendations. Put them in the same order as the basic cause so they will be easier to follow. If the recommendations call for work orders, purchase requests or other requirements, make certain that the information is carried forward to the Departmental Health and Safety Committee meeting for action and closing of the loop. All action items outstanding for longer than three months at the Departmental Health and Safety Committee meeting must be referred to the management policy forming committee for senior management action and follow up.

Make sure that you are familiar with the reporting and recordkeeping regulations in your area and that you abide by them.

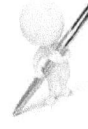

Activity 13:

13.1 Draw up procedures for your organization for recording incidents.

13.2 Draw up a sample of an incident report template.

SECTION 3 – FIRST AID LEVEL 1

Course Overview

First aid is the immediate skilled treatment of a person (s) at the scene of an injury or illness using available materials and resources available. It is the temporary assistance that is rendered until competent medical care, if required, arrives and takes over. An emergency is an unforeseen event or condition that requires a prompt response. This course is essential in the workplace and could save a life.

Course Outcomes

After you have completed this section you will be able to:

1. Demonstrate an understanding of emergency scene management.
2. Demonstrate an understanding of elementary anatomy and physiology.
3. Assess an emergency situation.
4. Apply First Aid procedures to the life-threatening situation.
5. Treat common injuries.

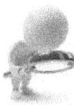

Go through the following table, this is an indication of what you will be expected to know and demonstrate an understanding in. Once you have completed this course return to this section and assess whether you grasp each specific outcome.

Specific Outcome	Assessment Criteria	Yes	No
1. Demonstrate an understanding of emergency scene management.	<ul><li>I am able to explain maintenance of personal safety is in terms of preventing injuries to self and infectious diseases.</li><li>I am able to explain methods of safeguarding the emergency scene in accordance with relevant practices and legislation.</li><li>I am able to explain methods of safeguarding the injured person in accordance with relevant practices and legislation.</li><li>I am able to explain the medico-legal implications of rendering First Aid in terms of relevant legislation.</li></ul>		
2. Demonstrate an understanding of elementary anatomy and physiology.	<ul><li>I am able to describe the different systems of the human body are in terms of their structure and function.</li><li>I am able to explain the manner in which the systems relate to each other in accordance with basic medical science.</li><li>I am able to explain the way in which each system operates in accordance with basic medical science.</li></ul>		
3. Assess an emergency situation.	<ul><li>I am able to assess the emergency situation in terms of priority treatments.</li><li>I am able to identify the cause of the emergency in terms of main contributing factors.</li><li>I am able to identify the type of injury in terms of broad classifications.</li><li>I am able to assess the situation in terms of the type of assistance required.</li></ul>		
4. Apply First Aid procedures to the life-threatening situation.	<ul><li>I am able to apply first aid treatment which is appropriate to the situation and the prevention of complications.</li><li>I am able to improvise equipment that is not readily available in terms of the First Aid procedure required.</li><li>I am able to take universal precautions which are appropriate in terms of preventing infection.</li><li>I am able to apply First Aid in accordance with current practice.</li><li>I am able to perform Cardio-Pulmonary Resuscitation (CPR) and Artificial Respiration (AR) in accordance with accepted procedures.</li><li>I am able to refer to medical assistance in accordance with the specific needs of the casualty.</li></ul>		
5. Treat common injuries.	<ul><li>I am able to identify and describe different types of injuries and conditions in terms of their severity, cause and possible treatment.</li><li>I am able to take universal precautions which is appropriate in terms of preventing infection.</li><li>I am able to improvise equipment that is not readily available in terms of the First Aid procedure required.</li><li>I am able to refer to medical assistance in accordance with the specific needs of the casualty.</li><li>I am able to follow-up care in accordance with the specific needs of the casualty.</li></ul>		

Definition of First Aid

First aid is the immediate skilled treatment of a person (s) at the scene of an injury or illness using available materials and resources available. It is the temporary assistance that is rendered until competent medical care, if required, arrives and takes over.

By applying first aid you are trying to achieve the following:

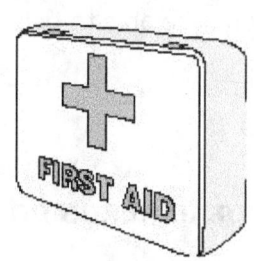

- Preservation of life (i.e. C.P.R.).
- Preventing the injury / illness from worsening
- Promoting the speedy recovery of the patient.
- Pain reduction.

Who is the First Aider?

The ideal FA is someone who is interested in the well-being of society. The FA also has very basic knowledge of the human body and has been trained to deal with situations to the best of their ability. The FA also puts in a concerted effort as well as regular self-evaluation of his / her skills.

The Role and Responsibility of the First Aider

The role of the FA has become a very important as the FA is a vital link between the time the incident occurs and the time the Emergency Medical Rescue Services (EMRS) arrive at the scene.

The responsibility of the FA is to:

- Assess the situation.
- Identify the problem / condition.
- Give immediate, appropriate and adequate treatment.
- Arrange transport.

The FA's responsibility ends once the patient is handed over to higher qualified help with a full report (history).

Emergency Scene Management (SO1)

An emergency is an unforeseen event or condition that requires a prompt response. In the event of an injury or medical emergency, a patient's health and / or life may very well depend on your ability react promptly, make a quick decision and render an appropriate level of first aid care until the emergency personnel arrives on the scene.

First aid personnel should be identified and summoned immediately to the scene.

Maintenance of Personal Safety

Your safety is the most important because if you are injured or killed then you will not be able to help the casualty and you will be adding to the problem.

"DEAD HEROS DO NOT SAVE LIVES"

All blood and certain body fluids that may contain blood should be considered potentially infectious, and precautions should be taken to protect you against them. No patient is to be treated **without** the protection of latex or vinyl gloves or one way valve because of the possibility of blood borne pathogens such as HIV/ AIDS and Hepatitis B transmission.

The Scene

The FA must learn to recognise potentially hazardous situations in cases such as:

- Road accidents - oncoming traffic, fuel spillage, unstable vehicles.
- Gas and poisonous fumes.
- Electricity lines.
- Fire and collapsing buildings.

Methods of Safeguarding the Emergency Scene

When you recognise an emergency, you must be prepared to take immediate action, preferably with an overall plan in mind. This plan must be one that occurs automatically. It should consist of basic steps that will help to establish control of the emergency scene. You must prepare yourself emotionally. Your own self-control may help to reduce the level of stress at the emergency scene.

The assessing and management of an emergency is the assessing of the scene, contacting of the EMRS and treatment of the patient (s).

On arrival first aiders should follow the procedure below:

Procedures	On arrival first aiders should follow the procedure below:
Step	Action
1.	Take charge of the situation.
2.	Call to attract the attention of bystanders.
3.	Assess hazards by establishing cause of accidents and secondary causes of the result of the accident.
4.	Identify yourself as a first aider and offer help.
5.	Before attending to the victim of any emergency, you must first survey the scene to ensure your safety.
6	Then, do a primary survey of the patient.
7.	After checking the victim, call the Emergency Services, giving them a description of the emergency situation as well as the location of the scene
8.	After calling the Emergency Services, provide appropriate care based on your primary survey of the victim until Emergency Services or other advanced medical personnel arrives and takes over

Primary Examination

The primary examination is done to determine any hazards at the scene and whether the patient(s) is has life threatening injuries/ conditions (i.e. Responsiveness and alive (breathing & pulse).

Assess Hazards

Assess the emergency scene for safety. Is it safe to approach the patient(s)? The safety of a scene must always be taken into account before entering the scene to minimise the risk to the first aider, the casualty and the bystanders.

ALERTING THE EMRS

WHEN SHOULD I CALL EMRS?

Respiratory Distress Signals:	Call EMRS if patient:
<ul><li>Breathing irregular.</li><li>Wheezing, gurgling or making high-pitched noises when breathing.</li><li>Short of breath, dizzy or light-headed.</li><li>Suffering from chest pain, tingling sensation in extremities.</li><li>Flushed, bluish in appearance or pale.</li><li>CALL EMRS.</li></ul>	<ul><li>Is or becomes unconscious.</li><li>Has chest pain or pressure.</li><li>Has difficulty breathing.</li><li>Is bleeding severely</li><li>Has pain or pressure in the abdomen.</li><li>Is passing or vomiting blood.</li><li>Has slurred speech, severe headaches or seizures (fitting).</li><li>Has a head, neck or back injury.</li><li>Has possible broken bones.</li><li>Has been poisoned.</li></ul>

Once you have assessed the scene and patient and decided that you require the EMRS, this information must be passed on to the EMRS accurately. This enables them to respond quickly and efficiently with the correct equipment and manpower.

WHAT NUMBER DO I USE?

Know the EMRS emergency numbers:

Local EMRS	10177 (Telkom) / 112 (Cell phone)
BLS Medical..	086 1178 243
NetCare 911...	082 911
ER24	084 124
SAPS	10111

WHAT DO I TELL THEM?

- Give the nature of the incident/ illness - when, who, how and give any complications.
- State your name & telephone number.
- Give the exact address/ location (use crossroads & landmarks).
- Give associated problems (fuel spillage, HAZMAT).
- Ask the EMRS operator's name.
- Answer any questions the EMRS operator may have and follow any instructions given by the EMRS operator.
- Put hand set down after the EMRS operator.

Methods of safeguarding the injured person

The Casualty

A casualty should never be moved from the scene unless remaining at that location is life threatening. Ideally, EMRS should respond to the scene. If life-threatening factors do exist by remaining at the scene, the FA should take extreme care not to cause further injury to the patient during the move. The spinal cord must be protected from any twisting or unnecessary movement during this effort.

It may be necessary to consider life over limb.

Patient Assessment

Patient Assessment is the gathering of information in a calm and systematic manner to establish whether the patient has:

- Any life-threatening conditions (primary survey) and
- Other injuries (trauma) and/ or medical conditions (secondary survey).

After completing a patient assessment you should have the following information available which will help in the treatment of the patient and with handing the patient over to higher qualified medical help.

S A M P L E - follow these helpful patient assessment steps prior to checking for the obvious problems.

S	**Signs and Symptoms**	What is the primary complaint? Check vital signs: • Skin Condition - Is skin red, pale, blue or yellow. Is the skin moist, clammy or dry? Hot, warm, cool or cold? Is the skin moist or pale? • Check level of consciousness - alert, unresponsive, confused, • Breathing - Is breathing rapid, slow, noisy? • Pulse - Is pulse rapid or slow? Strong or weak? • Eyes - Are the pupils of the eyes dilated (enlarged), constricted (very small), unequal (one pupil small, one pupil large) - PEARL?
A	**Allergens**	Ask patient about allergies to foods, medications, insects, or other things? Look for medical alert bracelets, necklace etc... Ask patient if they have been exposed to an allergen.
M	**Medications**	Is the patient taking any medication or under the influence of any drugs?
P	**Pre-Existing Medical History**	Look for medical alert bracelets, necklace etc... Ask the patient about any medical conditions that may relate to their current problems.
L	**Last Meal**	Ask the patient when they ate last and what did they eat?
E	**Events**	What events led up to illness or injury?

Critical Injuries

There are 3 injuries that take precedent over the rest and Emergency Services should be called if:

- The victim has sustained injuries to the head, neck or back;
- The victim is having trouble breathing;
- The victim is unable to move or use the injured body part without experiencing pain;

These require special and careful attention!!!!

The Medico-legal Implications of Rendering First Aid

During an emergency, the first aider can become involved in a variety of legal problems. You must however not be scared to treat someone because of the law.

The law will protect you from liability as long as you:

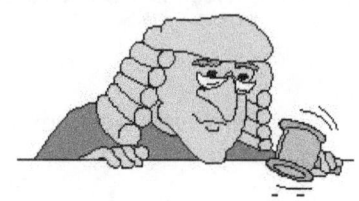

- Act in good faith.
- Are neither reckless nor negligent.
- Act as a prudent person would.

You must not abandon a victim once you have initiated care, and you cannot accept anything in return for your services.

There are certain aspects that need to be discussed.

PERMISSION (CONSENT)

No person may be touched without first giving his or her permission. Any person, who is touched or handled without permission, is considered to have been assaulted. This permission can be informed, implied or emergency (life threatening emergencies). It also must be remembered a patient may refuse you the right to treat them.

SCOPE OF PRACTICE

A FA may only treat a patient up to the level that he / she has been trained to. The FA certificate expires after 3 years, thus either a refresher needs to be done or a higher level.

DOCUMENTATION

The best way for a first aider to protect himself or herself against legal problems is good clinical documentation. Although the first aider is responsible for writing up detailed and sensible notes, there are no strict rules in this regard.

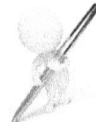

Activity 14:

14.1 Explain managing own personal safety at an emergency scene.

14.2 Discuss methods of safeguarding an emergency scene.

14.3 Discuss methods of safeguarding an injured person at an emergency scene.

14.4 Discuss the medico-legal implications of rendering First Aid.

Elementary Anatomy and Physiology

To be able to supply effective first aid, the FA must have a basic knowledge of the body and how it functions.

DIRECTIONAL TERMS

When dealing with a casualty, directional terms are described from the casualty's point of view.

- Right - Casualty's right and not the examiner's right.
- Left   - Casualty's left and not the examiner's left.

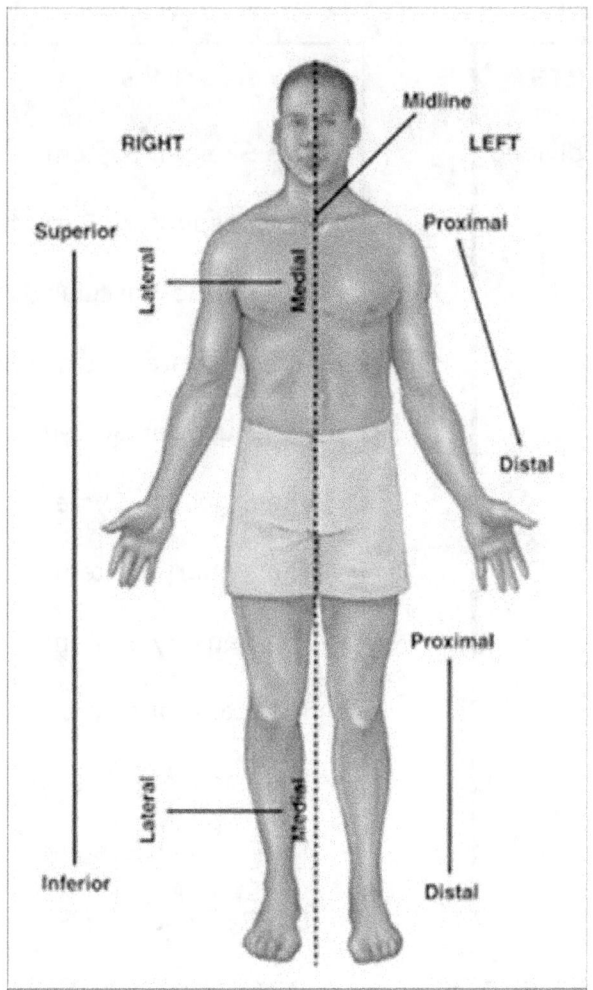

THE BODY REGIONS AND PARTS

The body as a whole, can be divided into 5 regions:

- The Head:
  - Cranium (Skull)
  - Face
  - Mandible (Lower jaw)

- The Cervical (Neck)

- The Trunk:
  - Thorax (Chest)
  - Abdominopelvic

- The Upper Extremities:
  - Arm
  - Wrist
  - Hand
  - Fingers

- The Lower Extremities:
  - Leg
  - Ankle
  - Foot
  - Toes

BODY SYSTEMS

- The Skeletal System

- The Respiratory System

- The Cardio-Vascular System

- Integumentary (Skin) System

- The Muscular System

- The Digestive System

- The Urinary System

- The Sensory System

- The Excretory System

- The Endocrine System

- The Nervous System

- The Reproductive System

CELLS, TISSUES, ORGANS AND SYSTEMS

Cells

A cell is the smallest building unit of the body. There are different cells in the body, each with its own specialised function; namely, nerve cells, muscle cells, sperm cells, blood cells, etc. Although cells vary in shape their structure remains the same with a nucleus surrounded by cytoplasm. Cells are continuously being replaced from a few days (skin cells) to a few years (bone cells). Each cell is a separate living organism and must be supplied with oxygen and nutrients by the bloodstream. If a cell does not receive oxygen it will die quickly. Irreparable damage can occur in **three to four minutes** in brain cells if they do not receive oxygen.

Tissues

A group of cells of the same type is called a tissue. Tissue fluids fill the spaces between the cells. The main tissues found in the body are: muscle 43%, fat 14%, organs 12%, skin 9%, blood 8%, etc.

Organs

An organ consists of the same type of tissues. An organ has a particular job to do in the body: the heart (pumps blood), stomach (digests food), eye (enables one to see), etc.

Systems

A system is a group of organs whose job is closely related. e.g. The circulatory system consists of the heart, blood vessels and to a lesser degree the bones of the skeleton which manufacture blood cells.

THE BODY CAVITIES

The body has many cavities but the most important two (2) are the dorsal and ventral cavities:

- Dorsal Cavities: This cavity is situated posteriorly and is divided into two smaller cavities.
  o Cranial cavity - Houses the brain and specialised membranes - Dura Mater, Pia Mater and Arachnoid.
  o Spinal cavity - Running through the centre of the back bone; protecting the spinal cord and its specialised membranes.

- Ventral Cavities: This cavity is situated anteriorly and is also divided into two smaller cavities.
  o Thoracic cavity - This cavity is subdivided again into smaller cavities which contain the heart (pericardial cavity), lungs (2 pleural cavities), major blood vessels, part of the trachea and oesophagus (mediastinum).
  o Abdominopelvic cavity - This cavity consists of two parts and is not physically separated. The abdominal cavity contains the liver, stomach, gall bladder, pancreas, spleen, small intestine and most of the large intestine. The pelvic cavity contains the bladder, large intestine and female reproductive organs. The kidneys are not found in the abdominal cavity but lie behind the peritoneal membrane (posteriorly).

THE ABDOMINOPELVIC QUADRANTS

The abdominopelvic region is divided into four quadrants and is named after their position, i.e. right and left upper quadrants and right and left lower quadrants.

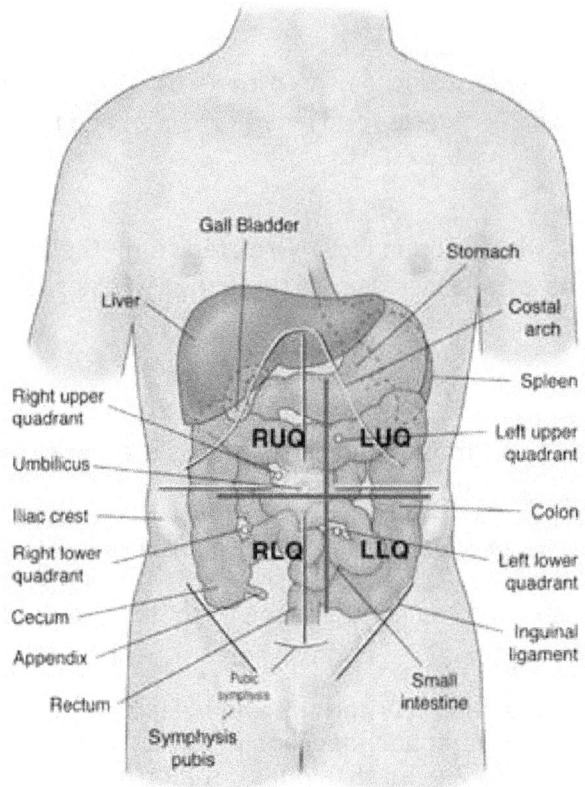

THE SKELETAL SYSTEM

The skeleton consists of 206 bones.

Functions of the Skeleton

- Protect the delicate organs.
- Framework and support - gives shape and rigidity to the body.

The Skeleton

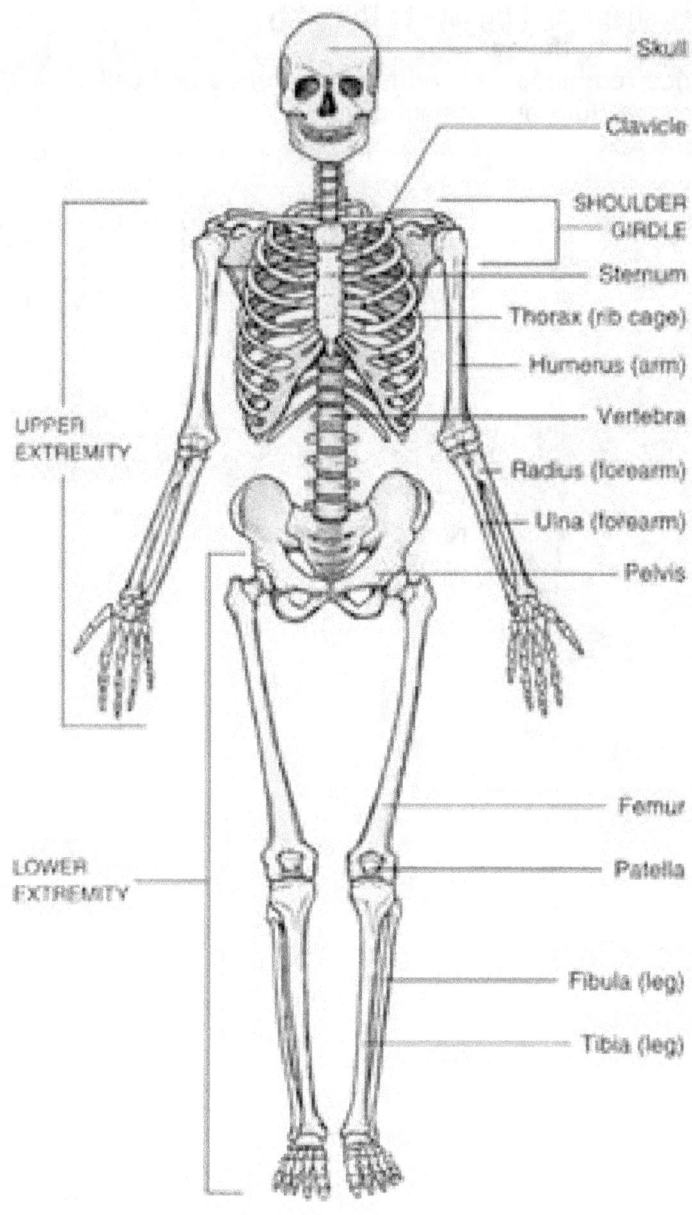

- Skull
- Clavicle
- SHOULDER GIRDLE
- Sternum
- Thorax (rib cage)
- Humerus (arm)
- Vertebra
- Radius (forearm)
- Ulna (forearm)
- Pelvis
- Femur
- Patella
- Fibula (leg)
- Tibia (leg)

UPPER EXTREMITY

LOWER EXTREMITY

Functions of the Skeleton

- Protect the delicate organs.
- Framework and support - gives shape and rigidity to the body.
- Aids in movement - muscles attach to bones.
- Marrow of certain bones produce red blood cells and some white blood cells.
- Storage place for minerals, esp. calcium and phosphorus.

The Cranium (Skull)

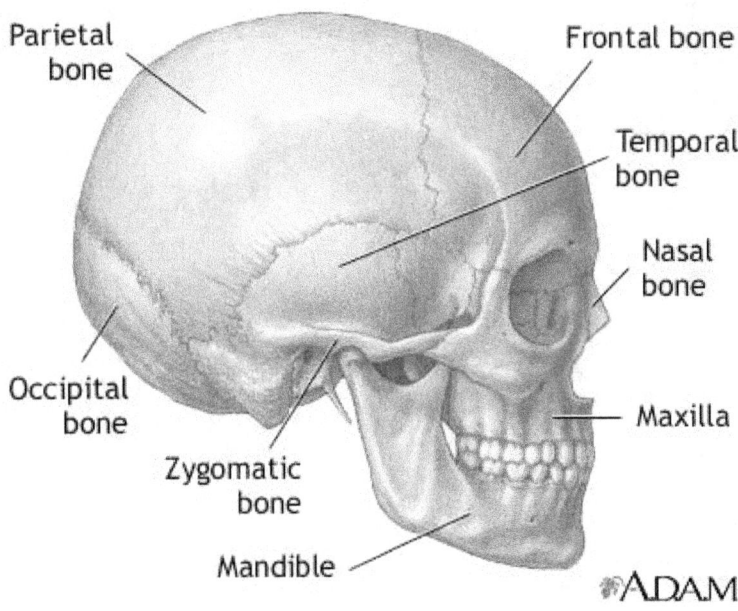

THE CRANUIM

The Spinal Column.

The spinal column consists of 33 vertebrae which are divided into:

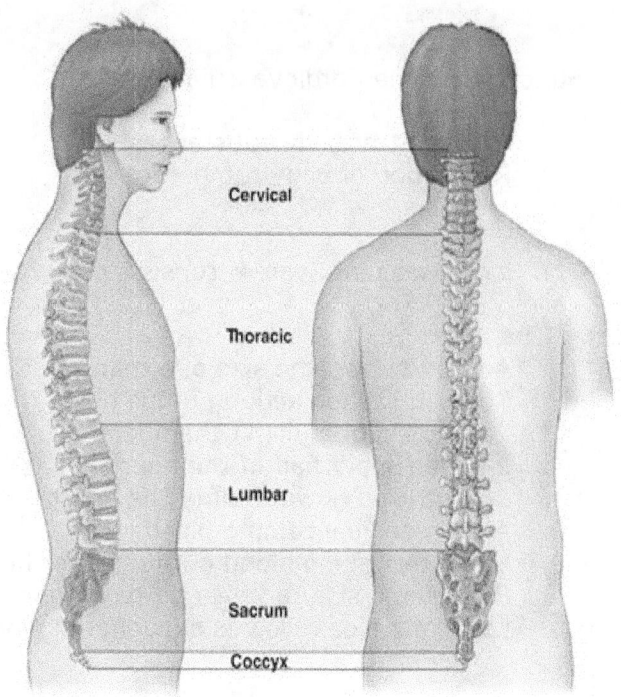

- **Functions of the Spinal Column:**
  - o Separate vertebrae form a column to protect the nerves.
  - o Allows movement in all directions.
  - o Forms a framework where other bones are attached and the cranium is carried by the spine.

The spinal discs act as shock absorbers (e.g. during the carrying of heavy objects).

The Pelvic Girdle

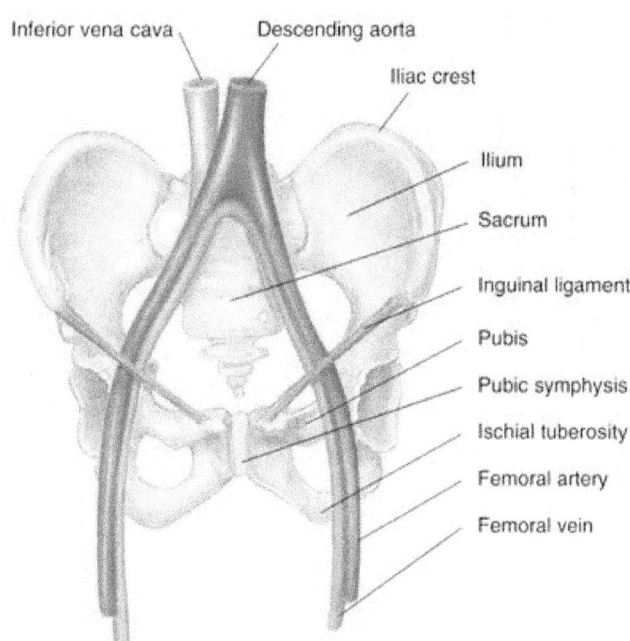

THE CARDIOVASCULAR SYSTEM

Functions of the Cardiovascular System:

- Transport of body substances.
- Regulation of body temperature.

The Cardiovascular System consists of:

- The Heart
  - Approximately the size of a man's fist.
  - The contraction action pumps blood through the body.
  - Comprises of four (4) chambers:
  - 2 Atria (upper half of the heart)
  - 2 Ventricles (lower half of the heart)
  - Atria receive incoming blood.
  - Ventricles pump blood out (stronger heart muscles).
  - Right hand side receives de-oxygenated blood, from the body and pumps to the lungs.
  - Left hand side receives oxygenated blood, from the lungs and pumps it to the body.

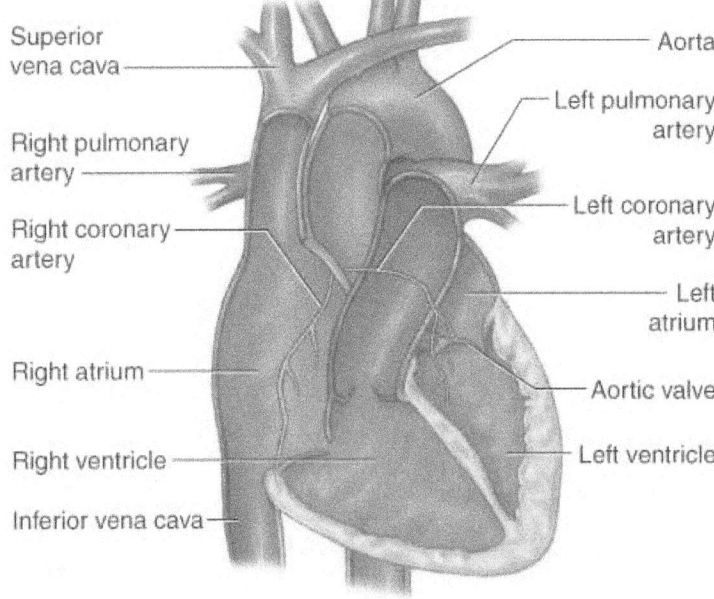

- The Blood Vessels
  - Arteries.
  - Capillaries.
  - Veins.

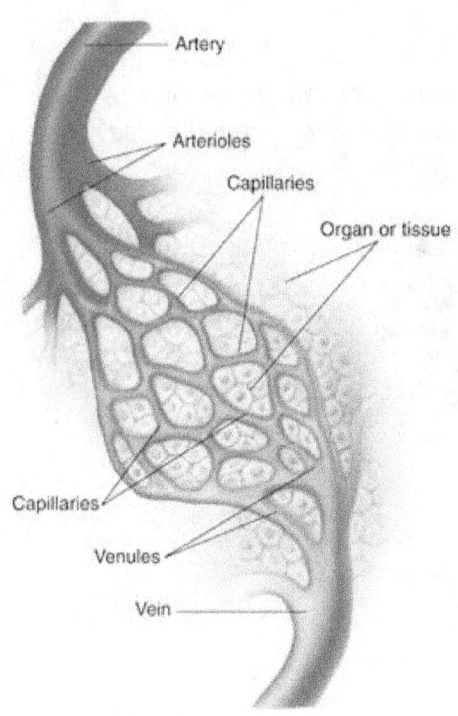

The Blood

The average adult has 71 ml / kg of blood in his / her circulatory system.

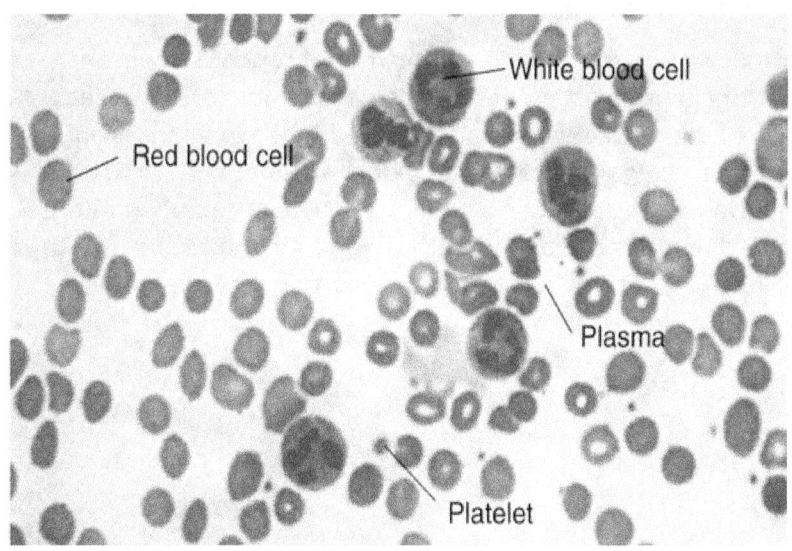

The Pulse

The ideal pulse for an adult is 60 – 100 beats per minute. It is usually felt for at one of the following places: the neck (carotid pulse) for unresponsive patients or wrist (radial pulse) for responsive patients.

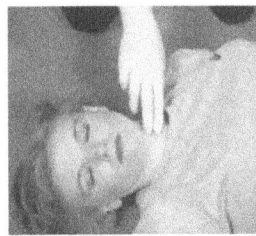 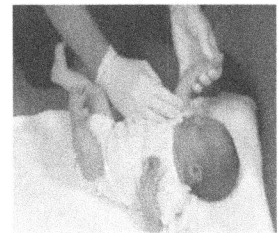 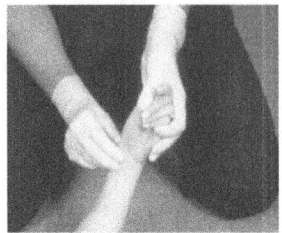

THE RESPIRATORY SYSTEM

Functions of the Respiratory System:

- To supply the body's tissue with vital oxygen.
- To remove waste gases from the body.
- Responsible for the ability to communicate.

Breathing

When one breathes in, air is passed through the nose and mouth and passes into the pharynx. The pharynx separates into two passageways, one being the oesophagus and the other the trachea. The trachea lies in front of the oesophagus.

From the trachea, the air enters the lungs through the left and right main bronchi. The bronchi tubes divide to smaller tubes called the bronchiole. At the end of these bronchiole are tiny sacs, called alveoli. The gas exchange takes place here with oxygen and carbon dioxide moving through the walls of the alveoli and capillaries. The oxygen enters the blood stream and circulates throughout the entire body feeding all the body's vital organs and tissue. Once the oxygen in the blood has been used, a by-product carbon dioxide is deposited in the blood for the return trip to the lungs. When the person exhales the unused portion of oxygen and carbon dioxide leave the body through the airway.

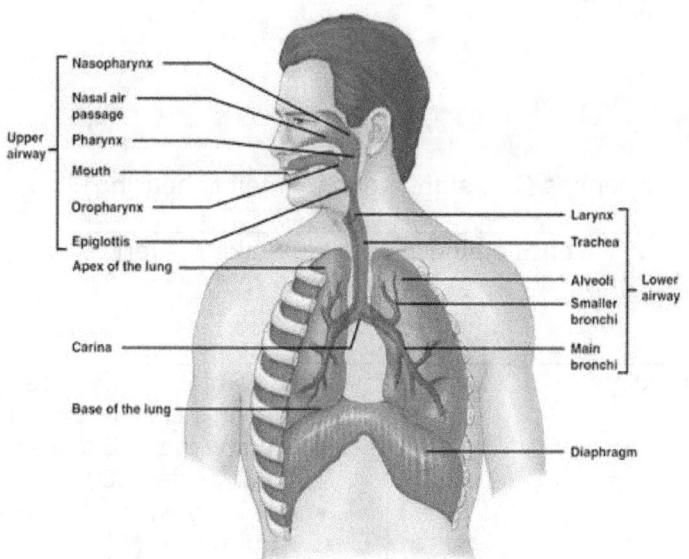

Typically, adults breath approximately between 12 - 20 breaths per minute (*1 breath every 5 seconds*) and children and infants 20 - 30 breaths per minute (*1 breath every 3 seconds*), under normal circumstances and is largely an automatic process.

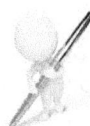

Activity 15:

15.1 Discuss the structure and functions of Cells, Tissue, and Organ System.

15.2 Discuss the structure and functions of the Skeletal System.

15.3 Discuss the structure and functions of the Cardiovascular System.

15.4 Discuss the structure and functions of the Respiratory System.

SIGNS

A sign is what you observe using your senses (i.e. sight, touch, smell & hearing).

Vital signs	Level of Consciousness (AVPU Scale)	• **A**wake & Alert. • **V**erbal. • **P**ain. • **U**nconscious.
	Skin Colour	• Grey-blue - (Cyanosis) - excess carbon dioxide. • Cherry-red - Excess Carbon Monoxide (CO). • Ash grey - Acute Myocardial Infarction (AMI).
	Skin Temperature & Moisture	(use the back of hand) - hot, cold, clammy or normal (37°C).
	Breathing	• Rate: Fast, slow or normal. • Quality: Deep, shallow or normal. • Regularity: Regular or irregular.
	Pulse	• Rate: Fast, slow or normal. • Strength: Strong, weak or normal. • Regularity: Regular or irregular.
	Pupils	• **E**qual **A**nd **R**ound, **R**egular (in size) and reacting to **L**ight **P**upils (PEARRL).
	Blood Pressure	110 -130/ 70 - 90 mm Hg.

Reassessment of The Vital Signs

The vital signs that you obtain serve two important functions. The first set is to establish a baseline of the patient's neurological, respiratory and cardiovascular systems and the quality of perfusion and oxygenation of the brain and other vital organs.

The second set is to determine whether the treatment that you are providing has restored the vital signs to an acceptable range or is at least preventing further deterioration.

In an unstable patient the vital signs should be taken and recorded every 5 minutes or after a medical intervention and with stable patients every 15 minutes.

Other Signs

- Bleeding: Type and volume.
- Fractures: Crepitus, deformity, swelling, bruising.
- Incontinence, vomiting, groans, reflexes, smell of breath (acetone).
- Needle marks, suspicious articles (OD's).
- Medic - Alert bracelet or medallion.

SYMPTOMS

A symptom is what the patient complains about.

Symptoms		
	Questions to ask the patient:	• What is wrong? • Where is the pain? • Are you allergic to anything? • Are you pregnant? - If female!
	Level of Consciousness - can be established by asking the patient:	• What is your name? • What day is it? • Where are you?
	Other Symptoms:	• Loss of feeling/ normal movement. • Nausea. • Fever

PROBLEMS WITH PATIENT ASSESSMENTS

- Type of injury:
  - More than one serious injury.
  - Severe traumatic injury which taxes the emotional stability of the first aider.

- Type of patient:
  - More than one.
  - Special (blind, deaf, dumb, drunk, uncooperative).

- Type of conditions:
  Dangerous (cross fire, fires, confined spaces, terrain).

  - Harsh weather conditions.
  - Uncomfortable environment (eg. small tunnel).
  - Uncooperative public.

ALERT

Hello

Identify yourself to the patient, bystanders or person in charge of the scene (e.g. I am John and a qualified first aider, may I help?).

Responsiveness

Try and determine if the patient is responsive (level of consciousness) (e.g. HELLO! Are you OK? Shoulder tap / sternal rub).

NO RESPONSE (UNCONSCIOUS)	RESPONSIVE (CONSCIOUS)
• Call EMRS.	• Introduction / request for consent.
• Check airway.	• Control bleeding if necessary.
• Check for breathing and circulation.	• Complete a head-to-toe exam.
• Provide CPR or rescue breathing, if necessary.	• Provide first aid if appropriate.
• Control bleeding, if necessary.	• Care for shock.
• Care for shock.	• Call EMRS if necessary.

Help

Call for help and try to get a bystander (s) to help you.

AIRWAY

Check the Airway

Check the airway for any visible obstructions. (Refer to the section on choking for the methods of clearing the airway).

If indicated, do a finger sweep or vomit roll.

Open the Airway

In the unconscious casualty the tongue often obstructs the airway. The following technique can be used to lift the tongue away from the back of the throat:

Head tilt - Chin lift (Pistol grip method).

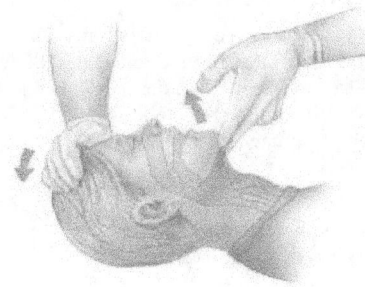

Place one hand on the casualty's forehead gently tipping the head backwards, at the same time placing the other hand on the chin in the pistol grip position (The forefinger along the jaw line, the thumb pointing in the same direction on top of the chin. The 3 fingers that are not used are curled up and placed under the chin.). The chin is then lifted slightly opening the airway.

OPENING THE AIRWAY – HEAD TILT CHIN LIFT

Maintaining the Airway

Keep the airway open by keeping the hand on the forehead in place.

BREATHING

Breathing is checked in the following way, for a minimum of 10 seconds:

LOOK - at the casualty's chest and abdomen for breathing movements.

LISTEN- for sounds of breathing.

FEEL - for airflow by placing your ear above the casualty's mouth and nose.

During checking for breathing you are trying to determine the following:

- **Normal Breathing.** The patient's chest and abdomen is moving, breath sounds can be heard and the exhalation of air can be felt on the check.
- **Respiratory Distress.** If a person is suffering from respiratory distress (dyspnoea - difficult breathing), they are not providing their body's tissues with enough oxygen. Some causes for respiratory distress include asthma, airway obstruction due to an object or allergic reaction, disease, and hyperventilation. (See page 8 for respiratory distress signs.)
- **Respiratory Arrest.** If a person stops breathing, it is called **respiratory arrest**. When a person stops breathing, the vital organs, such as the brain, heart and lungs can only continue to be oxygenated for a very short period of time. If the breathing stops, the respiratory system must be supported through rescue breathing (see below) before the heart stops (**cardiac arrest**).

If Respiratory Distress or Arrest is confirmed the First Aider must initiate Rescue Breathing (see below).

ASPHYXIA

Asphyxia is a potentially fatal condition due to the lack of oxygen (O_2) available in the blood. The body's tissues are dependant on the respiratory and circulatory systems to supply them with O_2. If one of the two systems fails, the body experiences a shortage of O_2 which can lead to permanent tissue damage.

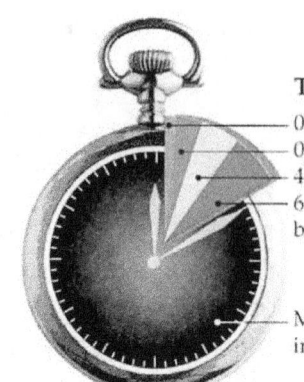

TIME IS CRITICAL!
0 to 1 minute: cardiac irritability
0 to 4 minutes: brain damage not likely
4 to 6 minutes: brain damage possible
6 to 10 minutes:
brain damage very likely

More than 10 minutes:
irreversible brain damage

CONDITIONS THAT CAN LEAD TO ASPHYXIA

- Smothering and insufficient oxygen in the air.
- Obstruction of the trachea.
- Compression of the airway.
- Compression of the chest.
- Fluid in the lungs (Drowning & Oedema).
- Lung contusion.
- Injuries that affect the respiratory and nervous system.

Signs and Symptoms

- Dyspnoea (difficult breathing).
- Inability to make verbal sounds.
- Universal distress signal.
- Cyanosis (bluish discolouration of the lips, tongue, mucosa, skin and nail beds).
- Exaggerated breathing.
- No sounds of breathing.
- Loss of consciousness.

Treatment
- Remove cause.
- Ensure airway is open.
- Ensure patient gets enough oxygen.

FOREIGN BODY AIRWAY OBSTRUCTION (CHOKING)

Respiratory emergencies, whether caused by a foreign body airway obstruction or as a result of illness or injury to any part of the respiratory system, are extremely distressful for the patient.

SIGNS AND SYMPTOMS

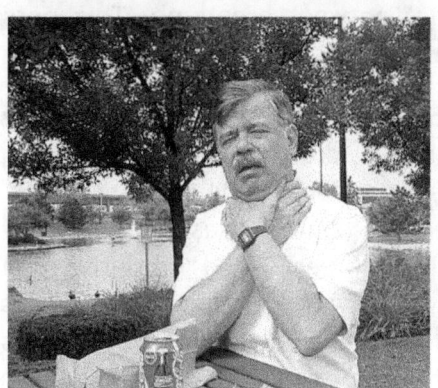

Partial Blockage

- Not a full expansion of the chest wall.
- Sounds during exhaling (whistling).
- Cyanosis.

Total Blockage

- No chest movement.
- No audible sounds.
- Unconsciousness.
- Cyanosis.

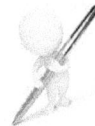

Activity 16:

16.1 Discuss the assessment process at an emergency.

16.2 Discuss prioritising treatments at an emergency scene.

16.3 Discuss causes of emergency and their contributing factors.

16.4 Identify types of injuries in terms of the following classifications:

Fractures	
Burns	
Lacerations	
Difficulty with breathing	
Severe haemorrhage	
Head injuries	
Spinal injuries	
Level of consciousness	
Strains and sprains	

CARDIO PULMONARY RESUSCITATION

During your assessment, you may have established that the patient is unresponsive (unconscious) and not breathing. This person is in **respiratory arrest and most likely in cardiac arrest**. This person needs CPR.

Whenever breathing and pulse stop, **"sudden death"** has occurred. "Sudden death" has many possible causes.... drowning, electrocutions, poisoning, choking, smoke inhalation, severe injury, but the most common reason is heart attack *(Acute myocardial infarction)*. "Sudden death" may be reversed in some cases. Rapid activation of EMRS combined with immediate CPR administration (if performed properly) can help a patient survive long enough to receive treatment with advanced medical techniques. CPR alone is not enough to save a patient's life in most cases of cardiac arrest. However, it is a necessary step within the chain of survival. By initiating and performing CPR, you are working to prolong the patient's opportunity to be brought back from "sudden cardiac death".

Your best chance to prolong brain activity through CPR is by alerting EMRS and starting CPR as soon as possible. Ideally, the EMRS should arrive and provide advanced cardiac care within 10 minutes. There is no time to waste once you recognise this emergency. EVERY SECOND COUNTS!

HOW CAN I TELL IF CPR SHOULDN'T BE STARTED?

CPR shouldn't be when there are positive signs of death are obvious to you. Do not start CPR.

WHAT ARE THE POSITIVE SIGNS OF DEATH?

- Rigour Mortis (body is extremely stiff and rigid).
- Tissue decomposition.
- Severe mutilation (e.g. Decapitation).
- Lividity (over time the lack of circulation results in pooling of blood on the down side of the body. Usually reddish-purple colour).

HOW DOES CPR WORK?

Once the blood is pumped into the lungs it picks up the oxygen and then goes to the rest of the body to deliver that oxygen. Without a heartbeat the oxygen cannot reach the vital organs.

The heartbeat is triggered by natural electrical impulses. The heart receives these electrical impulses 60 - 100 times per minute. Therefore, when cardiac arrest occurs, the first aider must simulate the heart's normal function. This is done by applying external cardiac massage or compressions. By compressing the chest, you are squeezing the heart between the sternum and back vertebrae, thereby forcing blood though the vital organs. Effective chest compressions only provide 25 - 33 % of the normal blood flow. Therefore, CPR is only effective in sustaining life for a short period of time.

CHEST COMPRESSION

- Place heel of dominant hand on the breastbone in the centre of the chest.
- Place other hand on top of the hand that is against the chest.
- Interlock fingers. Fingers should not be directly on chest.
- Your shoulders must be directly over your hands on the patient's chest.
- Lock your elbows.
- Compress breastbone 30 times to a depth of 4 - 5 cm, at a rate of 100 compressions per minute. Count aloud as you compress: 1 and, 2 and, 3 and,..... and 30.
- Allow complete recoil of the chest after each compression.
- Push smoothly without stopping at top or bottom.

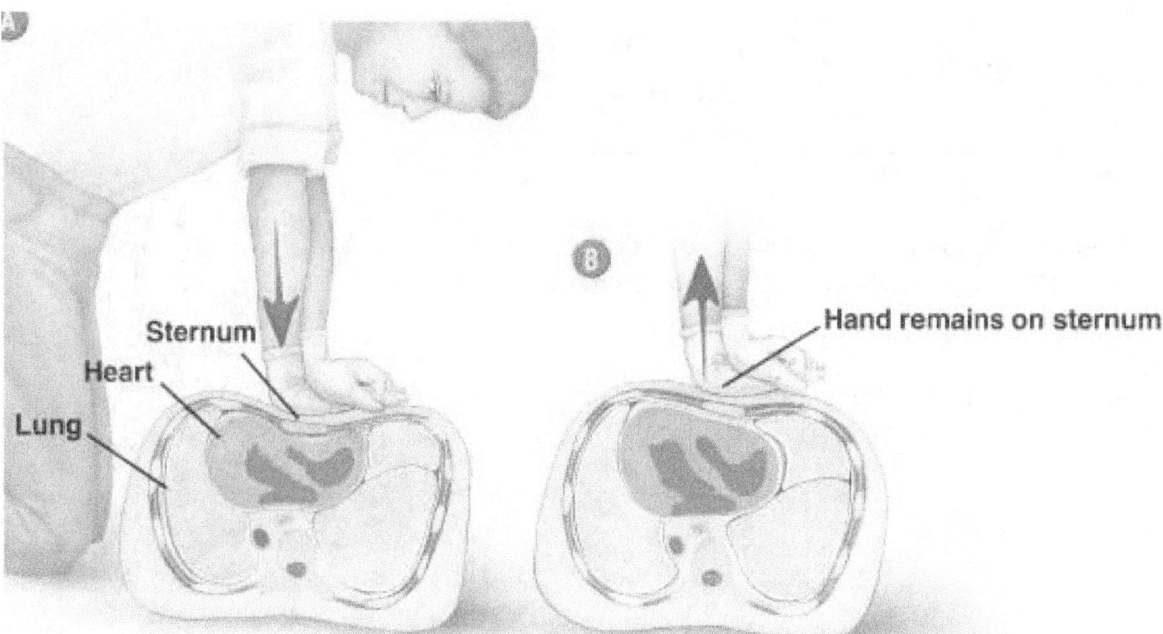

WHAT IF THE PATIENT VOMITS?

- Roll the patient towards you while supporting the head.
- Perform a finger sweep. Ensure the mouth is clear by checking.
- Reassess the patient.

HOW DO I KNOW IF MY CPR ADMINISTRATION IS EFFECTIVE?

- The chest will rise and fall with each ventilation.
- Have a second first aider check the pulse while you are doing compressions. If you are giving adequate compressions a pulse should be detected.
- The patient's colour should change as more oxygen is being given.

WHEN SHOULD I STOP CPR?

- When the patient begins to breathe spontaneously and there are signs of life.
- When qualified help takes over (i.e. Another first aider/ EMRS/ Doctor).
- When you are physically too tired to continue.
- It's too unsafe to continue, stop move casualty and then proceed once safe. CPR should not be interrupted for longer than 30 seconds.

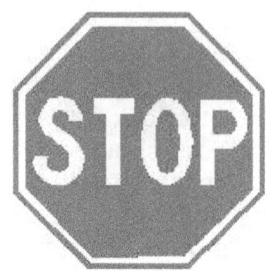

	CPR FOR AN ADULT OR CHILD **SUMMARY**	
1	**CALL** Check for Response. If no response, call 112 (cell) or 10177 for an ambulance (or other numbers as per page 25). Ask for CPR instructions if necessary.	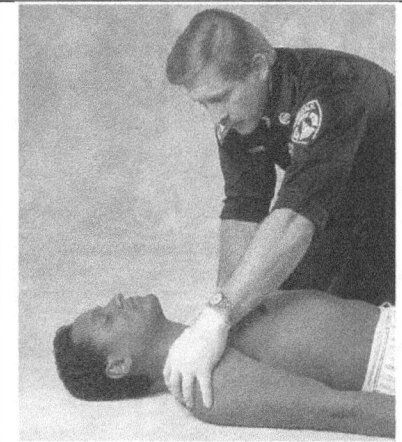 HELLO
2	**BLOW** Airway (check, tilt head back, lift chin up) and Breathing (look, listen & feel for breathing for up to 10 seconds). If Not breathing normally, pinch nose closed, cover mouth with your sand blow until you see chest rise. Give 2 breathes; each breath should take 1 second.	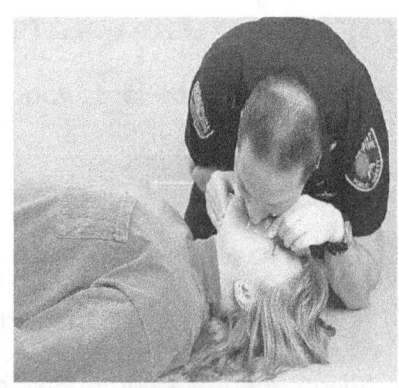 2 BREATHS

3	**PUMP** Give compressions by pushing down on the centre of the chest 30 times. Push hard and fast (almost 2 compressions per second). After 30 compressions give 2 breathes. Continue cycles of 30:2 until professional rescuers take over or normal breathing returns. Avoid interruptions.	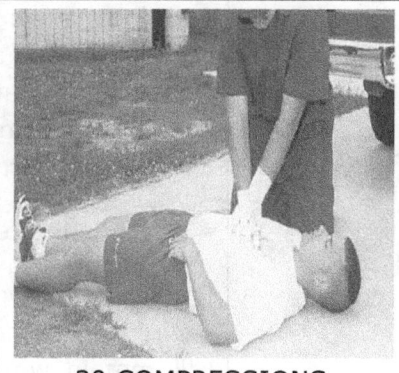 30 COMPRESSIONS

Types of Injuries/Illness in the Workplace

Bone Injuries/ Fractures	Your body consists of over 200 bones of all different shapes and sizes. All of these bones in addition to muscles and the tendons and ligaments that put them together form the skeleton, which serves to protect many of the organs your body uses to function normally. Bones are dense and very strong, and they tend not to break easily, except in elderly people who have developed osteoporosis, a gradual weakening of the bones. Bone injuries are often quite painful, and they may bleed, as all bones have an ample amount of blood and nerves.
	
	The two types of bone injuries are:
	
	    • **Fractures**, which may be open or closed, and
	    • **Dislocations**, which involve muscles and joints as well.
	
	An open fracture occurs when an arm or a leg twists in such a way that the broken bone ends tear through the skin, causing an open wound. In a closed fracture the skin is not broken; this type of fracture is much more common than an open fracture. An open fracture brings with it a chance of infection and also severe bleeding.
	Fractures can be life threatening if they sever an artery, affect breathing, or occur in very large bones such as the femur in the thigh. A motor vehicle accident or any fall from a height may cause a fracture.

Muscle Injuries	The body has over 600 muscles, which are soft tissue. Injuries to the brain, the spinal cord or nerves can affect a person's muscle control, and when a muscle is injured, a nearby muscle may take over for the injured one. A joint is formed where the ends of two or more bones come together in one place. The bones are held together by ligaments, which tear when a joint is forced beyond its normal range of movement.

	A dislocation is typically more noticeable than a fracture. A dislocation occurs when a bone moves away from its normal position at a joint. A violent force tears the ligaments that hold the bone in place at a joint and the joint will no longer function. Usually, the displaced bone causes an obviously abnormal bump, ridge or hollow. A sprain is the tearing of ligaments at a joint. Sprains may swell but typically heal quickly. Pain may be minimal and the victim may be active soon, in which case the joint won't heal properly and will remain weak. It is likely to be re-injured more severely, possibly involving a fracture or dislocation of the bones at the joint. The most easily injured joints are at the ankle, knee, wrist and fingers. A strain is a stretching and/or tearing of muscles or tendons. Lifting a very heavy object or working a muscle too hard frequently causes strains. They usually involve muscles in the neck, back, and thigh or back of the lower leg. Strains tend to reoccur; especially those located in the neck or back.

Burns	A burn can be caused by:
	
	   ✓ heat (flames, hot grease, or boiling water),
	   ✓ the sun (solar radiation),
	   ✓ chemicals or,
	   ✓ electricity.
	
	When a burn breaks the skin, infection and loss of fluid can occur. Burns can also result in difficulty breathing. If a burn victim has trouble breathing, has burns on more than one part of the body, or was burned by chemicals, an explosion, or electricity, call Emergency Services immediately.
	
	Burns caused by flames or hot grease usually require medical attention as well, especially if the victim is a child or an elderly person.

Sudden illness	The most common illness are: • heart attack • flu • shock • asthma • stomach ailments • allergic reactions Signs and symptoms of sudden illness include:

	- feelings of light-headedness; - dizziness, confusion, or weakness; - the victim may become pale or flushed, and may start sweating; - nausea and vomiting are causes for concern, as is diarrhea;	- changes in consciousness; - seizure paralysis; - slurred speech; - difficulty seeing; - severe headache; - breathing difficulty; - persistent pressure or pain;
	Call Emergency Services if: - victim has lost consciousness, is unusually confused, or is losing consciousness; - victim has difficulty breathing or is not breathing in a normal way; - has chest pain or pressure that won't go away;	- has persistent pressure or pain in the abdomen; - is vomiting or is passing blood; - has seizures, a severe headache, or slurred speech; - seems to have been poisoned; - has injuries to his/her head, neck, or back;
Head, Neck and Spine	These are considered critical injuries and take precedents over the rest and Emergency Services should be called.	
Shock	Shock is a life-threatening condition that can be caused by severe bleeding, an injury or sudden illness. The circulatory system fails to carry oxygen-rich blood to all body parts. The body's oxygen-starved major organs cannot function properly, triggering a series of responses, which produce specific signals known as shock. Three conditions are needed for the body to maintain adequate blood flow: - the heart must be working well, - an adequate amount of blood must be circulating, and - the blood vessels must be intact and able to adjust blood flow. When a severe injury or illness occurs, the body sends blood to the vital organs: - brain, - heart and - lungs, among others. When the tissues of the arms and legs begin to die, the body sends blood to them and away from the vital organs.	

	The victim goes unconscious as the brain is affected, his or her heartbeat slows and stops as the heart is affected, and then breathing stops as well. **Without proper medical treatment, a person in shock will die.**
Fainting or a diabetic emergency	When the insulin level in the body is too **low** and the blood sugar level is too **high**, the resulting condition is called **hyperglycemia**. If this condition is not corrected, the victim may go into a diabetic coma. When the insulin level in the body is too **high** and the blood sugar level is too **low**, the resulting condition is called **hypoglycemia**.

Bone injuries/fractures

Procedures	To care for bone injuries or fractures, proceed as follows:
Step	**Action**
1.	Do not try to move a patient with a severely broken bone unless it is absolutely necessary.
2.	Calling Emergency Services is the best course of action in this case.
3.	However, if you must move the patient you must immobilize the injured body part. One way is to splint it, but do this only if it can be done without hurting the victim, and always attempt to splint the part in the position you found it.
4.	Splint the injured area & the joints above and below the injured area. You may use another body part, like an injured leg to an uninjured one, or an injured arm to a chest - this is called an *anatomic splint*. Make a *soft splint* from folded blankets or towels, or use a triangular bandage to make a sling, another type of soft splint, which is used to support an injured arm, wrist or hand. Use folded magazines or newspapers, cardboard or metal strips to support the injured body part with a *rigid splint*. Use several folded triangular bandages to secure the injured body part to the splinting material, tying them securely but not too tight.
5.	Apply ice and raise the injured part, and prevent the victim from getting chilled or overheated.
6.	Remember to be reassuring!

Muscle Injuries

Procedures	To care for a muscle injury, proceed as follows:
Step	**Action**
1.	The formula for proper care is rest, ice and elevation.
2.	Make the victim as comfortable as possible, and apply ice to reduce pain and swelling.
3.	Minimize movement of the injured part by supporting it with something like a pillow.

Burns

Procedures	To care for burns, proceed as follows:
Step	**Action**
Thermal Burns	
1.	Stop the burning. Put out flames or remove the victim from the source of the burn.
2.	Cool the burn. Use large amounts of cool water to cool the burn. Never use ice except on small superficial burns, because it causes body heat loss. If the area cannot be immersed, like the face, you can soak a clean cloth and apply it to the burn, being sure to continue adding water to keep the cloth cool.
3.	Cover the burn. Use dry, sterile dressings or a clean cloth to help prevent infection and reduce pain. Bandage loosely. Do not put any ointment on a burn unless it is very minor. Do not use any other home remedies, and do not break any blisters. For minor burns or burns with broken blisters that are not severe enough to require medical attention, wash the burned area with soap and water, keep it clean and apply an antibiotic ointment. Remember that some people can be allergic to topical ointments, so if you have any doubts, call your doctor for advice. For a victim of severe burns, lay him or her down unless he or she is having trouble breathing. Try to raise the burned areas above the level of the victim's heart if possible, and protect the victim from drafts.
4.	Chemical burns can be caused by chemicals used in manufacturing or in a lab, or by household products such as bleach, garden sprays or paint removers.
5.	Call Emergency Services in any case of a chemical burn.

6.	Remove the chemical from the skin or eyes immediately by flushing the area with large amounts of cool running water until Emergency Services arrives. Remove any clothes with chemicals on them, and be careful not to spread the chemical to other body parts or to yourself.
Electrical Burns	
7.	Electrical burns can be caused by power lines, lightening, defective electrical equipment, and unprotected electrical outlets.
8.	Call Emergency Services in the case of an electrical burn.
9.	Do not go near the victim unless you are sure the power source has been turned off.
10.	The burn itself will not be the major problem.
11.	If the victim is unconscious, check breathing and pulse.
12.	Check for other injuries, and do not move the victim because he or she may have spinal injuries.
13.	Cover an electrical burn with a dry, sterile dressing. Do not cool the burn.
14.	Prevent the victim from getting chilled.
15.	There may be two wounds, one where the current entered the body and one where it left, and they may be deep.

Head, Spine, Neck Injuries

Procedures	To care for head, spine or neck injuries, proceed as follows:
Step	**Action**
1.	If in a victim you see these signs: • changes in consciousness; • vision and breathing problems; • nausea and vomiting; • inability to move a body part; • steady headache; • tingling or loss of sensation in hands, fingers, feet or toes; • blood in the ears or nose; • seizures; • severe pain; • pressure or bleeding in the head, neck or back; • bruising of the head; • loss of balance;

	Call Emergency Services immediately, and **DO NOT** attempt to move the victim or you may injure him or her further.
2.	Minimize movement of the head and spine, maintain an open airway (lift the chin slightly but **DON'T** tilt the head otherwise you might paralyze the victim),
3.	Check consciousness and breathing,
4.	Control any bleeding,
5.	Prevent the victim from getting chilled or overheated.

Cuts

Procedures	You will need: soap, hot water, cotton wool or gauze swabs, antiseptic lotion, plasters or a non-adhesive dressing (clean tissues will do) and a gauze bandage, then proceed as follows:
Step	**Action**
1.	Wash your hands.
2.	Press the wound with thumb and fingers (holding cut edges together if necessary) until bleeding stops.
3.	Rinse wound under a tap if it's dirty,
4.	Then, using cotton wool or gauze, gently clean with soap and water. Work from the centre of the wound outwards, using a clean swab for each wipe.
5.	Finish with some diluted antiseptic.
6.	Pat skin thoroughly dry.
7.	Carefully remove any small pieces of glass or gravel from the wound with a clean piece of gauze tweezers.
8.	For small cuts and grazes, a plaster is enough.
9.	Larger injuries need a non-adhesive dressing secured with a gauze bandage which you tie firmly, but not so tightly that the circulation is restricted.
10.	**Never** put fluffy dressings like cotton wool next to the wound – they'll stick to it and it will be painful when it comes to pulling it off. Only handle the very edges of a dressing.

Shock

Procedures	To care for shock, proceed as follows:
Step	**Action**
1.	Call Emergency Services immediately.
2.	Have the victim lie down in order to rest comfortably, minimizing pain.
3.	Control any bleeding.
4.	Prevent the victim from becoming chilled or overheated.
5.	Reassure the victim.
6.	Elevate the legs about a foot unless you suspect head, neck or back injuries or broken bones in the hips or legs, in which case you must leave the victim lying flat.
7.	Do not give the victim anything to drink.

Fainting or a Diabetic Emergency

Procedures	To care for fainting or a diabetic emergency, proceed as follows:
Step	**Action**
1.	If you know that a person is diabetic and he or she is experiencing these symptoms, treat the person as though he or she has hypoglycemia, or low blood sugar.
2.	If the victim is conscious, give him or her something to eat or drink that contains plenty of sugar, such as sweets, fruit juice, cola, etc. If the person is suffering from low blood sugar, or hypoglycemia, the sugar will help within minutes. If the person is feeling ill because of high blood sugar, or hyperglycemia, he or she will not be harmed by the extra sugar.
3.	If the victim does not feel any better after five minutes, call Emergency Services.

Sudden Illness

Procedures	To care for a sudden illness, proceed as follows:
Step	**Action**
1.	First, call Emergency Services immediately and care for any life-threatening conditions the victim may have.
2.	Help the victim rest comfortably, and prevent him or her from getting chilled or overheated.
3.	Reassure the victim. Monitor him or her for changes in consciousness, and do not give the victim anything to eat or drink unless he or she is fully conscious.
4.	If the victim **vomits**, place the victim on his or her side to prevent choking.
5.	If the victim **faints**, position him or her on the back and elevate the legs about a foot if you do not suspect a head, neck or back injury. A person about to faint becomes pale, begins to perspire, and then loses consciousness and collapse. Remember the adage: "if the head is pale, raise the tail," which refers to returning blood and circulation to normal after fainting.
6.	If the victim has a **diabetic emergency**, give him or her some form of sugar drink or sweet.
7.	If the victim has a **seizure, DO NOT** place anything in his or her mouth. Remove any nearby objects that might injure the victim. Cushion his or her head with a pillow or folded blanket, towel or article of clothing. Move yourself out of the victim's range as he or she will probably be thrashing violently and you do not want to be injured. After the seizure, keep the airway clear and place the victim on his or her side if there is fluid, like blood, saliva or vomit, in his or her mouth.

AILMENTS	SYMPTOMS	TREATMENT
Appendicitis	Pain in right lower abdomen. Nausea, possible vomiting and fever.	Call your doctor. Never give anything by mouth. Ice back may reduce discomfort.
Burns & Scalds	Redness & pain. Moderate burn will blister. Severe burn shows tissue destruction.	Ice for small burn. Cool (not ice) water to big burn. Wash with cool water & soap. Sterile dressing. NO ointment. Do not remove clothing stuck to burn. Call a doctor if extensive, blistered, or white, dry and painless.
Convulsions	Strong, jerking movements; stiff body. Difficulty breathing. Bluish face. Eyes rolled back, gritting or teeth, frothy mouth.	Call doctor. Prevent patient from hurting himself. Keep them lying down, do not restrain. Loosen collar, and cover him.
Croup	Noisy, difficult breathing. Hoarse, barking cough.	Call you doctor. Expose immediately to moist air; use a humidifier in a small room or put patient in the bathroom and turn on the shower (keep door and windows closed).
Dog Bite	Skin may be punctured or torn. May show teeth/fang marks.	Wash with soap and water, cover with sterile dressing and bandage. Capture animal to observe for rabies. (If must kill, preserve head for rabies tests). Report to a doctor or hospital.
AILMENTS	SYMPTOMS	TREATMENT
Drowning	Unconscious, not breathing. Heart may have stopped.	If victim has pulse but no breath, give mouth to mouth breathing. If heart stopped, give CPR – if trained. DO NOT move head, neck or back unnecessarily. Call ambulance.
Electric Shock	Unconsciousness. Pale, bluish skin that is clammy and mottled in appearance.	Turn off current, break contract with dry wood or dry cloth. If no breath, give mouth to mouth. If no pulse, give CPR (if trained). Keep patient warm. Give nothing to eat or drink.

Fractures & Dislocations	Severe pain, deformity, and loss of motion. Possible protruding broken bones.	Call doctor. Do not move injured part until splinted. If legs, back, neck are injured, keep person lying flat and call ambulance. Cover open wounds with available clean fabric. Keep patient warm. Give nothing to eat or drink.
Gas Poisoning	Headache. Dizziness. Pale. Unconscious.	Open or smash windows and doors, pull victim to fresh air. If no breath, give mouth to mouth. If no pulse, give CPR (if trained). Keep warm. Call ambulance.
Heat Stroke Exhaustion	**Heat Exhaustion:** Pale, clammy, headache and weakness. Possible nausea. **Heat Stroke**: also vomits, is flushed and confused.	Cold cloths to skin. Give salty fluid such as broth, Gatorade or Pedialyte. If patient vomits or becomes flushed and confused, he has **Heat Stroke**! Call ambulance or doctor.
Heart Attack	Persistent chest pain, often radiating to left shoulders and arms. Difficulty breathing. Lips, skin and fingernails turn blue.	Call an ambulance. Place victim in a comfortable position, sitting up. Use pillows for support. Keep warm and loosen collar. If trained, administer CPR (if trained), otherwise give mouth to mouth resuscitation if breathing has stopped. Give nothing by mouth.
Poisoning	Symptoms vary. Throat or stomach pains. Mouth burns. Vomiting. Drowsiness.	Call Poison Centre or a doctor. If directed, give syrup of ipecac. DO NOT force liquids or induce vomiting unless so directed.
Shock	Due to injury, illness, poison: pale, mottled face, cold sweat, fast breathing, weak pulse.	Keep warm, lying down, feet raised. Call a doctor or ambulance. No fluids or food. Clear airway. If lower face/jaw injuries, or unconscious: lay on side to drain. Avoid rough or excessive handling.
Stroke	Unconscious. Heavy breathing. Apparent weakness in face or limbs on one side. Inability to speak.	Cover patient with a light blanket. Turn head of vomiting patient to side. Give no stimulants and nothing to eat or drink. Call an ambulance.

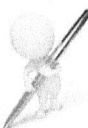

Activity 17: Discuss treatment for the following injuries.

Fractures	
Burns	
Lacerations	
Difficulty with breathing	
Severe haemorrhage	
Head injuries	
Spinal injuries	
Unconsciousness	
Strains and sprains	

MANAGING SHOCK, BLEEDING AND OTHER CIRCULATION EMERGENCIES

Care for shock is standard treatment in all first aid related emergencies. Shock is a condition in which the cardio vascular system fails to provide adequate blood circulation to all parts of the body for perfusion of oxygen. When the body's organs do not receive an adequate supply of blood, they fail to function properly.

In a minor injury, the body will compensate and this situation will be resolved in a short time. In the case of more severe injuries, the body may not be able to adjust. If the body cannot adjust or compensate for blood or other body fluid loss, shock will occur.

SIGNS AND SYMPTOMS

- Skin - pale, cold and clammy.
- Level of Consciousness - decreases from conscious to unconscious.
- Respiration - Rapid, shallow, sighing, air hunger.
- Pulse - initially rapid and strong to rapid and weak.
- Eyes - dull, pupils dilated.
- Thirst.
- Nausea and vomiting.
- Anxious, restlessness or irritability.

TREATMENT

W	Warmth - Maintain the casualty's body temperature.
A	Airway - Ensure that the casualty gets enough fresh air and/ or oxygen.
F	Fluids - Nil per mouth.
E	Elevation/ Positioning (This depends on the casualties' injuries). - Raise the legs 20 - 30 cm above the ground. - Recovery position (unconscious patient). - Semi-sitting for respiratory or cardiac conditions. - Flat on the back (spinal injury).
R	Reassurance.

UNCONSCIOUSNESS

Unconsciousness is a condition where there is a decrease/ loss of mental awareness and the body's ability to react to stimuli.

LEVELS OF CONSCIOUSNESS

Alert: Aware of surroundings.

Verbal: Aroused with verbal commands/ questions.

Pain: Responds to severe painful stimuli.

Unconscious: No reaction to any stimuli.

CAUSES OF UNCONSCIOUSNESS

There are many causes of unconsciousness and it is not possible to consider all of them. The FA must know the most common causes so he/she can pick up specific signs and symptoms.

Cause	Possible Clues, Signs and Symptoms
Head injuries	Visible signs and symptoms. Mechanism of injury.
Overdose	Medicine containers or syringes and syringe needles. Vomitus with visible medication. Empty bottles and a smell of alcohol.
Diabetes	Insulin and syringes. Needle marks. "Medic-Alert". Fruity smell on the breath (green apple).
Convulsions	Bitten tongue. Loss of bladder control. Medication. Bystanders.
Stroke	Asymmetry of the face. Weakness or paralyses on one side of the body. Medication for hypertension.

NB. The state of unconsciousness of an individual is probably the single most reliable sign in the assessing the status of one's nervous system.

TREATMENT

- Determine the cause of unconsciousness,
- Treat the injuries found (if any),
- Place the patient in recovery position, if no spinal injury
- Monitor and reassure the casualty.

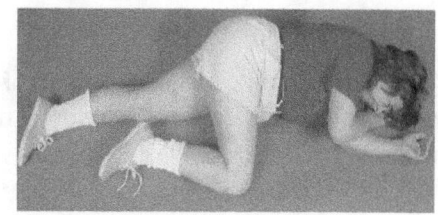

RECOVERY POSITION

WOUNDS

Wounds can be categorised as follows:

OPEN WOUNDS

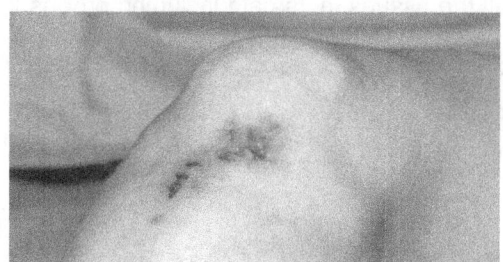

Abrasions - Scrapes and scratches; outer layer of skin is damaged (e.g. skid on rough ground).

Incision - Smooth, clean cut with a sharp object (e.g. knife). Often there is profuse bleeding, and sometimes stitches (sutures) are required.

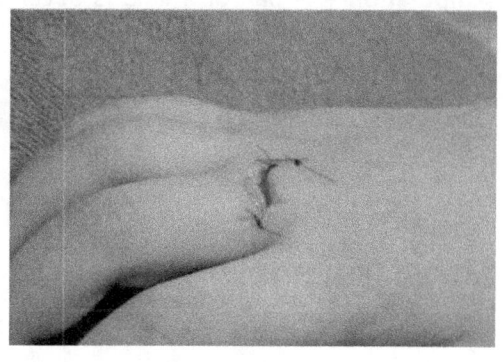

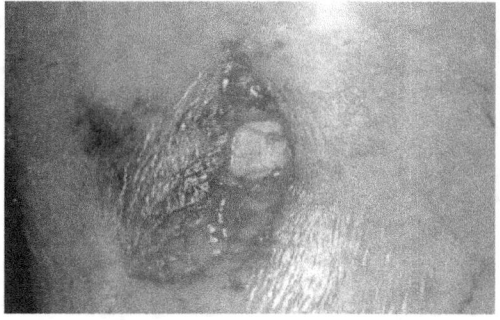

Laceration - Jagged cut. Heals very quickly as the edges of the wound are irregular and the blood clots can attach themselves with ease.

Avulsion - It is a wound where part of the soft tissue forms a flap. (e.g. ear partially torn / ripped from the head).

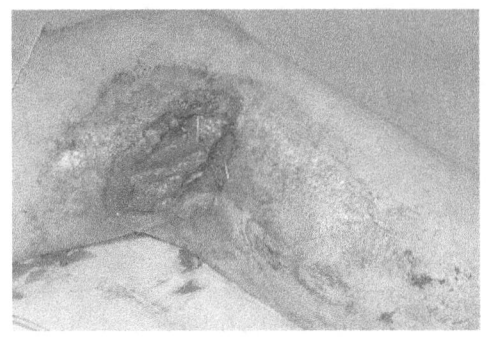

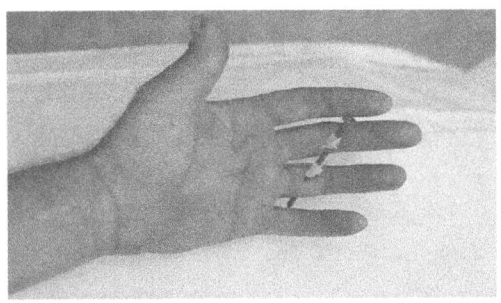

Puncture - The object passes through the skin and damages all the tissues in its path including organs if penetration is deep enough. It may pass through the body and cause an exit wound (e.g. stabbing, gun shot and bite wounds).

Amputation – A part of a limb is severed from the body.

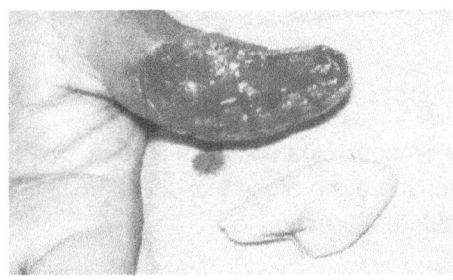

CLOSED WOUNDS

Contusion – Bruise – Skin surface is not broken but blood vessels under skin are ruptured, resulting in blood leaking into the surrounding tissue.

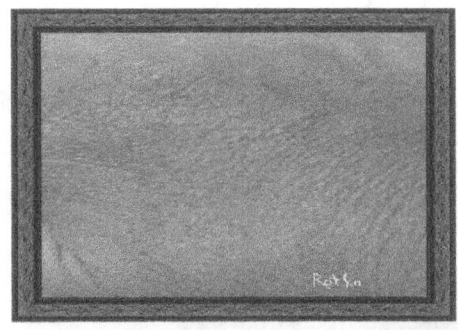

BLEEDING EMERGENCIES

Bleeding (haemorrhage) means that blood is escaping from the cardiovascular system from the arteries, veins and/ or capillaries.

It is estimated that the average adult's body holds approximately 71ml/kg of blood. The rapid loss on more than 750 ml or more can lead to shock and death. A child losing more than 450 ml of blood is in danger. Severe Bleeding must be brought under control.

CLASSIFICATION OF BLEEDING

Arterial Bleeding

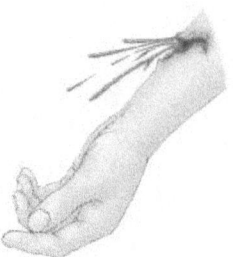

The opening of an artery results in the most serious type of bleeding. When blood is released from an artery, it is oxygen rich and will look bright red. The flow will often spew forth in rhythmic spurts that coincide with the hearts contractions. If a major artery is cut and not treated promptly, it is possible to bleed to death in as little as one minute.

DANGER ! DANGER ! Follow bleeding control sequence and activate the EMRS immediately!

Capillary Bleeding

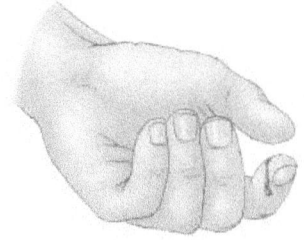

The capillaries are the smallest and most numerous blood vessels in the body. When a cut or scrape opens capillaries, typically the bleeding will be slow. Your body should be able to control this bleeding through its own blood clotting ability. Rarely will you have a rapid or uncontrolled loss of blood in this situation.

First Aid for Minor Wounds with Minimal Bleeding:

- Remove clothing covering the wound,
- Clear the surface of the wound (wash all loose dirt away),
- Clean wound with water and soap and then apply antiseptic (clean from inside the wound outwards),
- Apply a clean dressing to prevent infection.

Venous Bleeding

This is usually the result of a deep cut that opens veins. This will release blood that its way back to the heart. The blood from this wound will be dark red. It flows steadily. If left untreated, a life-threatening condition may result. **You must control this bleeding.** If bleeding persists after you have provided bleeding control first aid, sutures will be needed.

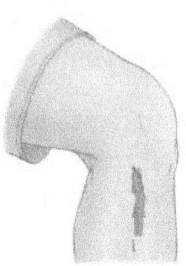

Transport to medical centre or call EMRS.

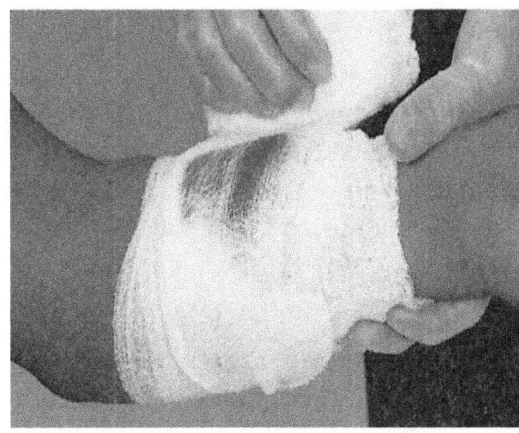

APPLYING A MATERIAL BANDAGE

	The Bleeding Control Sequence	
1		**Direct pressure** At this time, a direct pressure bandage may be applied.
2		**Elevate** Do no further harm.

THE BLEEDING CONTROL SEQUENCE

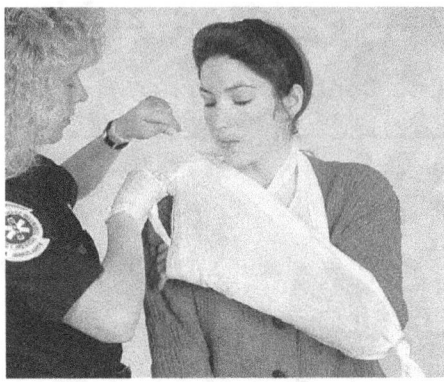

Internal Bleeding

Internal bleeding may not be visible. The signs vary depending on the nature, volume and cause of the bleeding.

Signs and Symptoms:

- Bleeding from one of the body's orifices (nose, ear, mouth, rectum, and urethra),
- Bruise or contusion,
- Signs and symptoms of shock,
- Nausea and vomiting,
- Painful, tender or hard spot on abdomen or chest,
- Puncture or penetrating wounds,
- Fractures.

First Aid Care:

- Care for shock,
- Watch for vomiting,
- Apply ice pack to injured area, place cloth between ice and skin,
- Call EMRS!

Impaled (Foreign) Object

An impaled object can be anything from a piece of glass, metal, wood, shrapnel, knife or even a fractured bone (open fracture) sticking out of a wound.

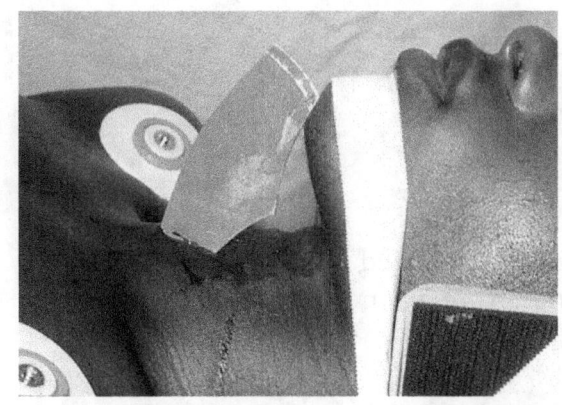

Do not remove the object!! Control bleeding as best as possible without disturbing the object. Stabilise the object with a ring or roller bandages. Restrict the patient's movements.

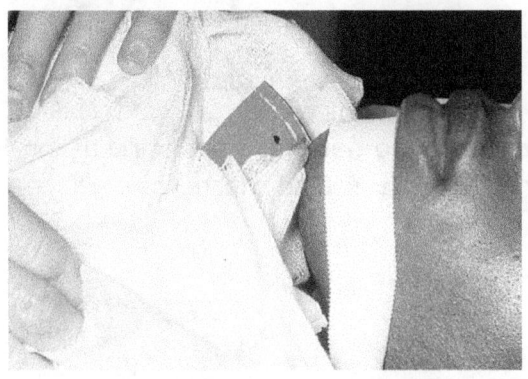

STABILISATION OF AN IMPALED OBJECT, USING ROLLER

BANDAGE.

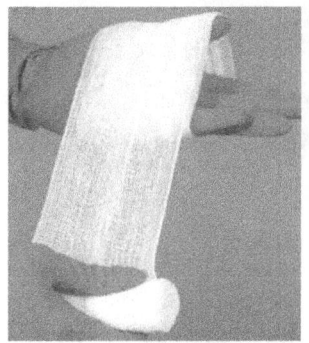
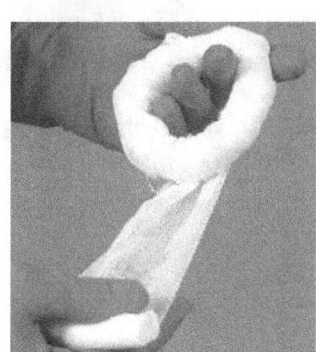
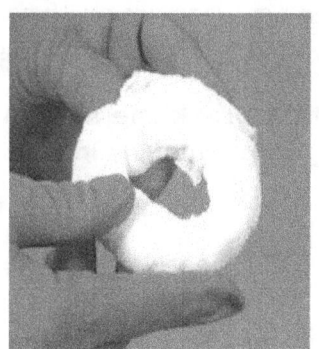

MAKING A RING BANDAGE

Scalp and Face Injuries

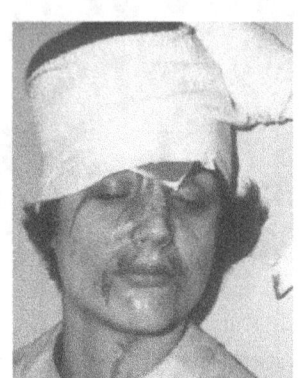

The head and face is rich in blood supply thus these injuries bleed profusely even though a major blood vessel may not have been severed. Follow *Bleeding Control Sequence*.

Amputation / Severed Body Part

Follow *Bleeding Control Sequence*. Do not scrub body part. Do not place part directly on ice. Wrap part in a sterile or clean cloth. Place part or cloth in a sealed plastic bag. Place bag containing part on a bed of ice. Do not bury in ice.

Bites (Animal / Human)

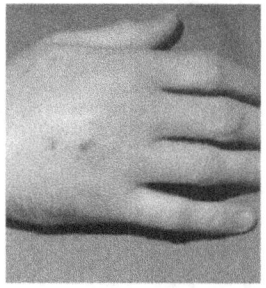

Control bleeding. Clean area with soap and water for at least 5 minutes. Cover the wound with a sterile dressing. **Seek medical attention for**

any bites that break the skin. Any human or animal bites <u>may cause infection.</u> A tetanus immunization may be recommended.

Infection

An injury that breaks the skin can lead to infection. Common symptoms include wound area becoming hot, red, swollen and painful. Wound may discharge pus. Red streaks may develop near wound. Victim may become ill and feverish. Seek medical attention for persistent or severe infection. A tetanus immunisation can help the body fight tetanus bacterium.

Restrictive Bandages

Once the bandages have been placed the circulation below the bandages must be monitored to determine if the blood circulation has been affected. Common signs and symptoms would be the part distal to the bandage will feel cold; the patient will complain of feeling pins and needles in the part distal to the bandage and the limb will be pale or blue-grey.

The treatment is quite simple and that is to restore blood circulation by applying the bandage more loosely.

EYE INJURIES

Eye injuries are generally not life threatening. They can, however, be severely detrimental to the patient in the long term.

Foreign Objects (penetrating or superficial)

The eye will appear:

- Eye - watery and red.
- Scratchiness in the eye.
- Foreign object visible in the eye when the eyelid is pulled up or down. The eyelids are opened using the thumb and forefinger.

Treatment

Foreign Objects in the Eye (Non Penetrating)

- Explain the treatment to the patient before starting.

- Rinse with clean non-irritant liquid (water, milk etc.).
- If the object is seen use wet gauze or soft tissue paper remove it.
- Should the object not be easy to remove, cover both eyes with gauze swabs kept in place with plaster.

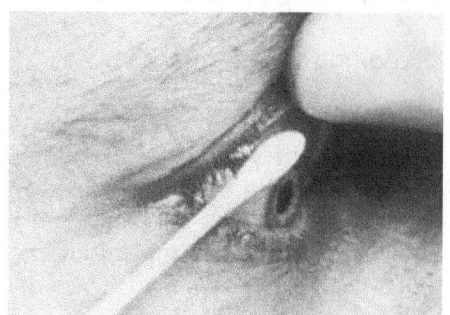

Penetrating Wounds of the Eye

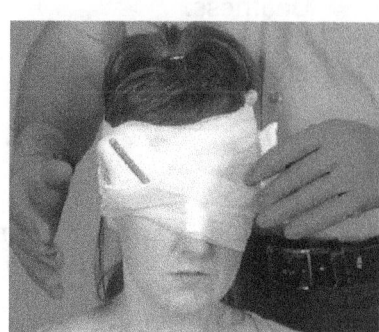

- Should the object of penetration still be in place, do not remove or disturb!
- Protect the eye by placing a roller bandage or ring pad around the object.
- Place a paper cup or cone over the object to prevent it from being disturbed.
- Bandage other eye without applying any pressure to the eyeballs.
- Do not use any ointments or eye drops.
- **SEEK MEDICAL ATTENTION!**

Chemicals in the Eye

Flush eye with water immediately for at least 15 – 20 minutes continuously.

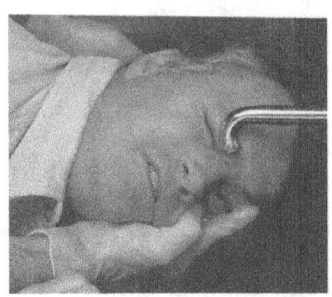

- Roll Eye as much as possible during flushing to assist washing the chemical out.
- If only one eye is affected, rise contaminated eye downward away from other eye.

Cuts or blows to the Eye

- Patch both eyes. **SEEK MEDICAL ATTENTION!**

EAR INJURIES

Ear injuries usually occur from pressure being put onto the tympanic membrane (ear drum) or from head injuries.

Signs and Symptoms

Bleeding from the ear (s):

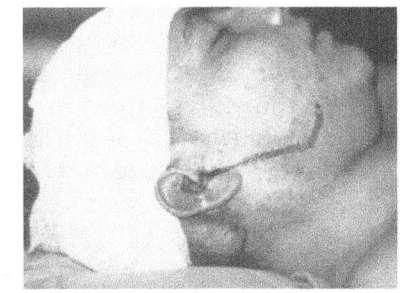

- o Possible base of skull fracture, if accompanied with a head injury and/ or headaches. The blood can be combined with a straw coloured watery fluid (cerebro-spinal fluid - CSF) that trickles from the ear.
- o Ruptured tympanic membrane - a small quantity of blood flows from the ear.

- Deafness.
- Pain – throbbing.
- Loss of balance.

Treatment

- Ruptured ear drum *(tympanic membrane)* - Tilt the head to the injured side for drainage.
- Suspected base of skull fracture - *Treatment as for Neck-Spine Injuries* .
- Cover the ear with a sterile dressing (Do not plug the ear).
- Should the pinna (external ear) be damaged it should be placed in the correct position and kept in place by a bandage.

NASAL INJURIES

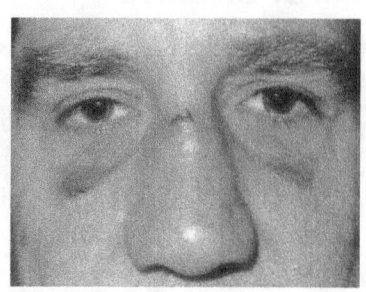

Nasal injuries and bleeding are caused by various factors, namely: fractures, blows to the face, high blood pressure, blood diseases, high temperatures and climate.

Signs and Symptoms

- Bleeding from the nose:
  - Ruptured blood vessel - bright red blood.
  - Possible base of skull fracture, if accompanied with a head injury and/ or headaches. The blood can be combined with a straw coloured watery fluid (cerebro spinal fluid) that tickles from the ear.
- Discolouration around eyes (Racoon eyes/ Peri-orbital Bleeding).

Treatment

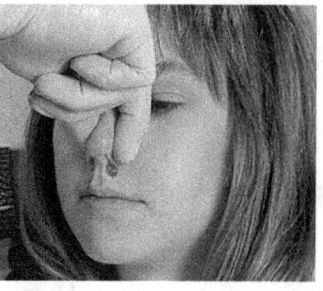

- Ruptured blood vessel:
  - Tilt the head forward and pinch the soft part of the nose below the nasal after 30 minutes seek medical aid.
  - An ice pack can be placed on the bridge of the nose and on back of neck.
  - Advise the patient not to cough or blow his/her nose.
- Suspected base of skull fracture. Do not stop the bleeding. Use gauze swabs only to absorb the blood. –
  Treatment as for Neck-Spine Injuries

CHEST INJURIES

Open Chest Wounds

Open chest wound without a penetrating object - Cover the wound to prevent outside air from getting into the chest cavity. You can use plastic to place over the opening. Leave one corner untapped as this will prevent air from being taped in the chest but allow any trapped air to escape from the chest.

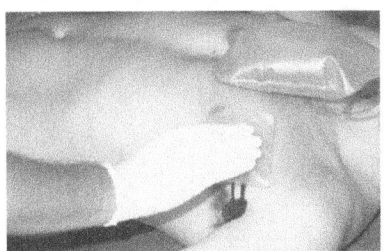 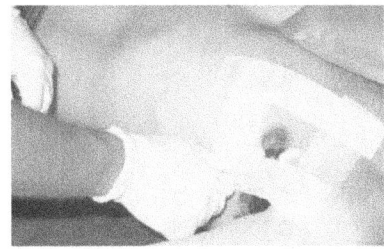 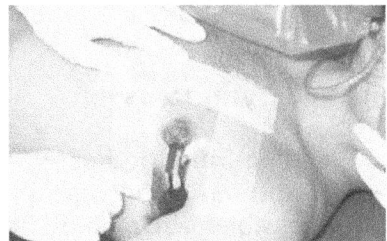

COVERING AN OPEN CHEST WOUND

Closed Chest Wounds

Closed chest wound caused by a blow to the chest area - Have patient hold a pillow against injured area. Watch for signs of shock because there may be internal bleeding. **SEEK MEDICAL ATTENTION!**

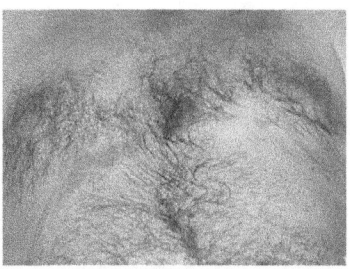

ABDOMINAL INJURIES

Always suspect internal damage and bleeding. Call EMRS and provide care for shock. Never touch protruding organs. Always cover the organs with a wet, sterile dressing. Use a bandage to keep the dressing in place, without applying pressure to the protruding organs. If available cover the dressing with plastic and secure all four sides with plaster. Place the casualty in the most comfortable position (i.e. On his/her back, legs bent.) And be prepared for vomiting.

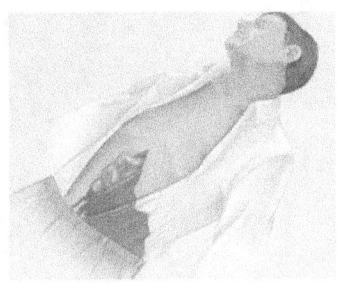 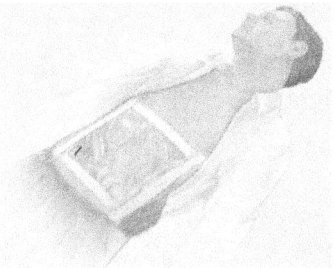

COVERING PROTRUDING ORGANS

MANAGING FRACTURES, HEAD AND SPINAL EMERGENCIES

Fractured bones and dislocated joints can be extremely painful, and debilitating. If not treated correctly, a more serious condition can result.

Head and spinal injuries are often treated as a result of the mechanism of injury, and may lead to possible permanent paralysis.

FRACTURES AND DISLOCATIONS

A fracture is a break in the continuity of bone tissue whereas a dislocation occurs when a joint is forced out of its normal position and remains in that position...

CLASSIFICATION

Closed - A fracture/ dislocation occurs without a break in the skin surface. It can however still become an open fracture/ dislocation.

Open - A fracture/ dislocation is in contact with the atmosphere (the surface of the skin is broken).

SIGNS AND SYMPTOMS

- History of trauma (snapping sound).
- Pain.
- Swelling and discolouration.
- Deformity.
- No or limited movement.
- Shortening of the limb involved.
- Exposed bone.
- Abnormal movement.
- Irregularity of the skin surface.
- Tenderness.
- Crepitus (grating sound).
- Loss of distal pulse.
- Loss of sensation.
- Muscle spasm

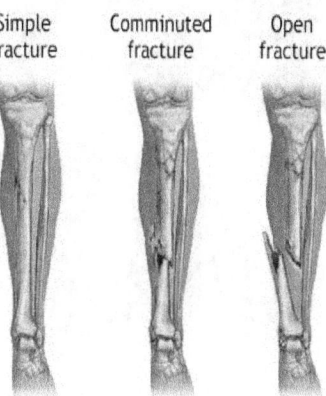

Simple fracture   Comminuted fracture   Open fracture

ADAM.

TREATMENT

I	**Immobilise area** • Immobilise - splint above and below the fractured site and the joints. • Stabilise and cover any protruding bones with sterile dressing (Ring bandages). • Check distal pulses and nerve function (sensation & motor) again.
A	**Activate EMRS** (or transport patient to a medical centre)
C	**Care for Shock**
T	**Treat any additional secondary injuries**

* If EMRS response time is questionable or you decide to transport, it is recommended that you splint the injured area. This will enhance the immobilisation and reduce the risk of additional injury.

DISLOCATION INJURIES

Dislocation injuries must **never** be replaced / repositioned!

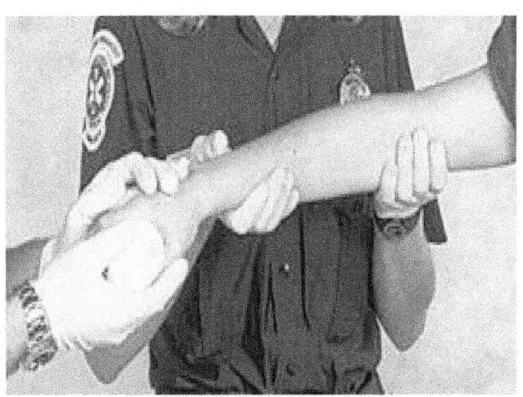
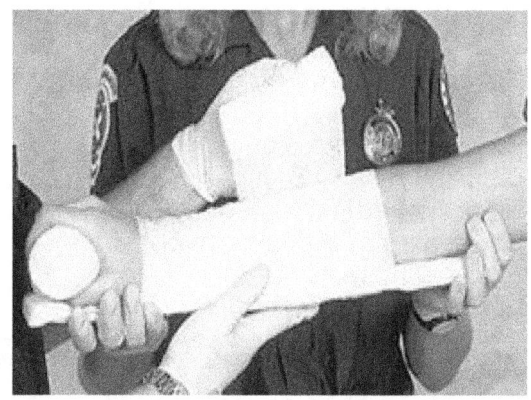

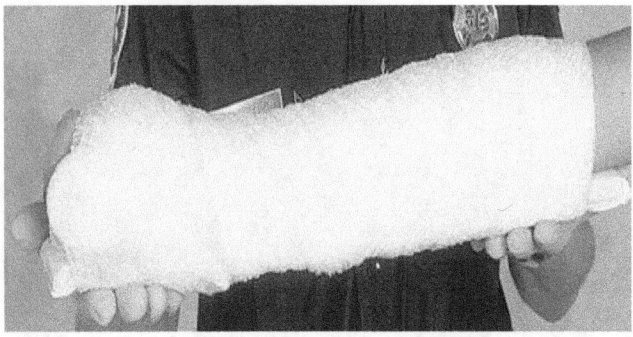

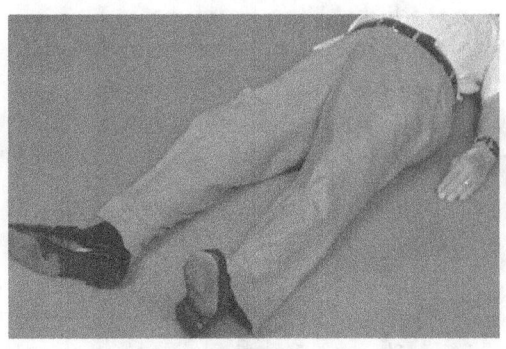
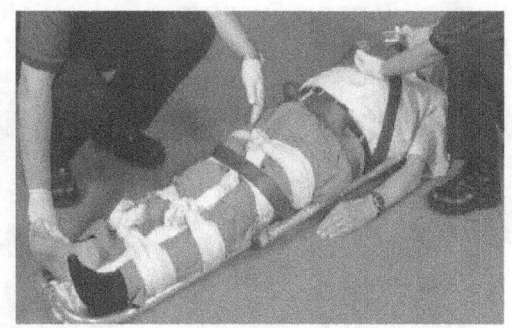

SPLINTING A FRACTURED LEG BONE USING THE BODY AS A NATURAL SPLINT

VARIOUS TYPES OF SPLINTING

Splinting of a Femur Fracture	Splinting of a Ankle Fracture
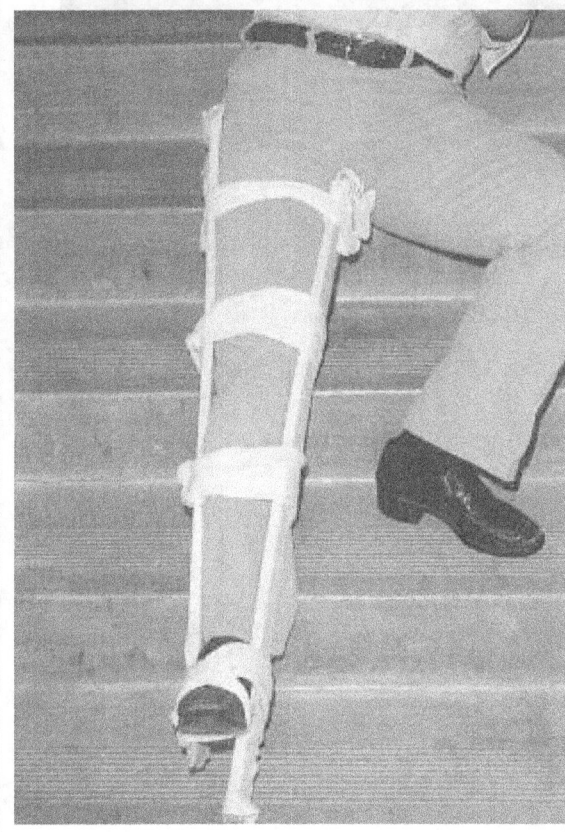	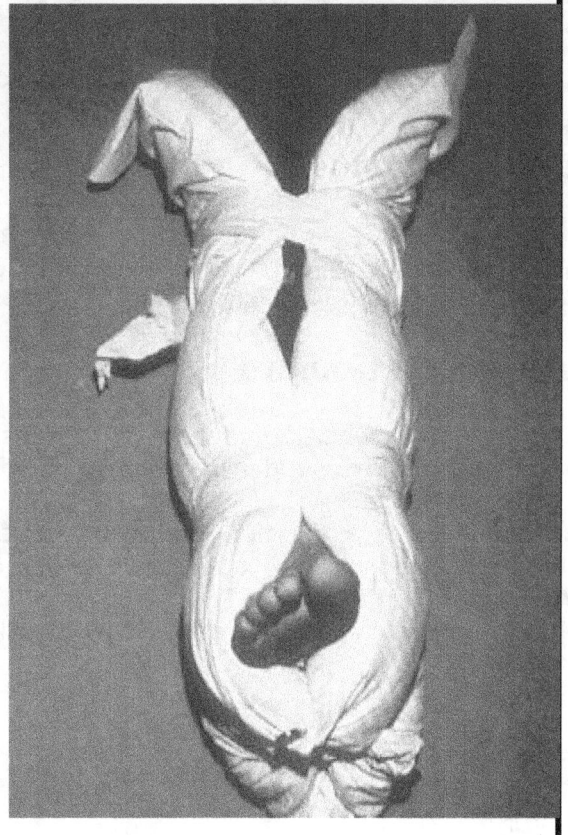

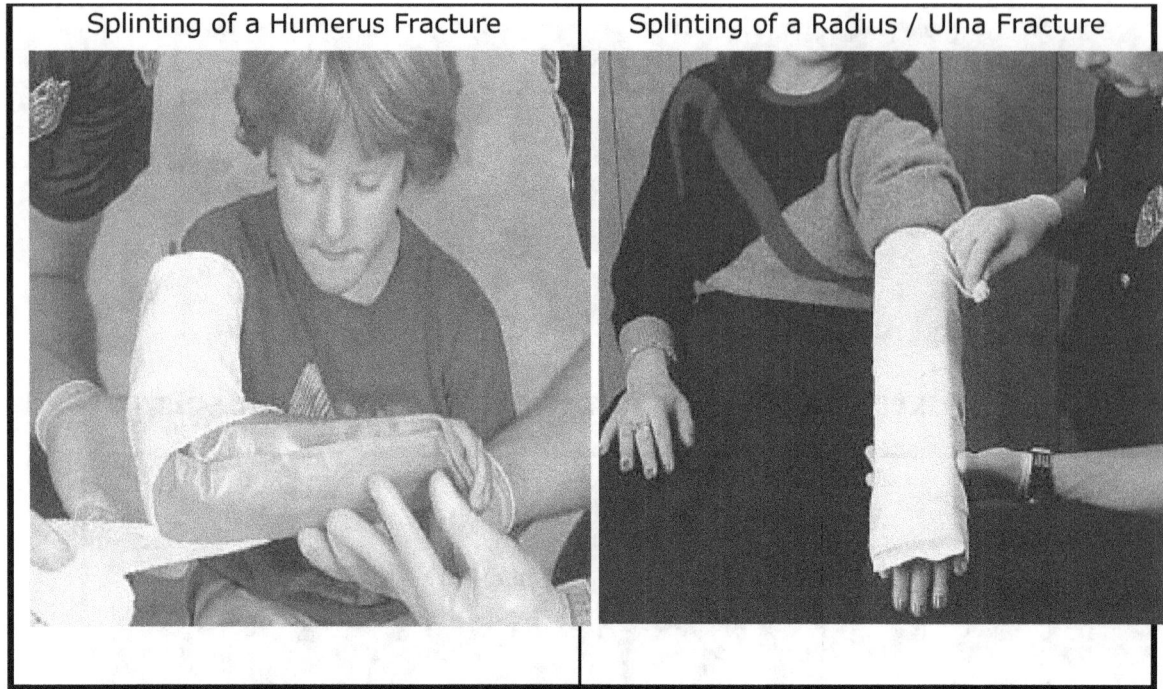

| Splinting of a Humerus Fracture | Splinting of a Radius / Ulna Fracture |

SPRAINS AND STRAINS

An injury to the body's musculoskeletal system requires immediate care. Any unnecessary movement should be avoided. Prompt first aid may reduce trauma and accelerate healing. If you are not sure of the severity of injury, treat it as a fracture or dislocation.

TYPES OF MUSCLE INJURIES

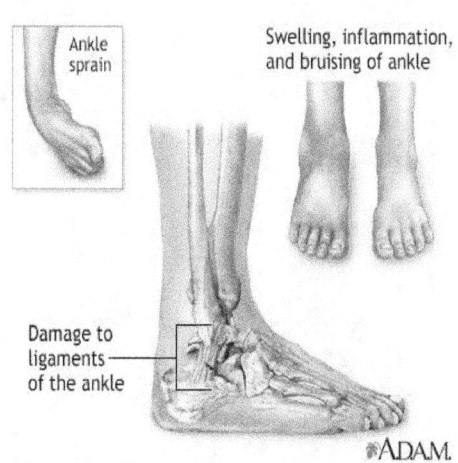

- Sprains occurs when ligaments and tissues around a particular joint are suddenly stretched or torn beyond its normal range.
- Strains is when a muscle/ group of muscles is over-stretched and possibly torn by a violent or sudden movement.
- Muscle Contusion results from a blow or a knock to a muscle.

SIGNS AND SYMPTOMS

- History
- Pain on movement
- Swelling
- Discolouration
- Limited movement.

TREATMENT

General First Aid for Sprains, Strains and Contusions		
R	**R**est Discontinue activity.	
I	**I**ce Apply a cold pack. Do not place ice directly on skin.	
C	**C**ompression Bandage Use an elastic or conforming bandage to hold the ice in place initially. Apply support to joint by using figure-8 bandage.	
E	**E**levate The injured limb above heart level to control swelling and any internal bleeding.	

HEAD, NECK AND / OR SPINAL COLUMN INJURIES

The central nervous system forms the main controlling system of the body and can be damaged quite easily. Any injury or illness that affects this system must be handled with extreme caution and care. The spinal cord runs through the centre of the spinal column, and is thus easily susceptible to injury. The cervical and lumbar vertebrae are often damaged, e.g. in whiplash injuries and by incorrect lifting of heavy objects.

You must always suspect head or spinal trauma when the patient has been injured as a result of:

- Motor vehicle accidents.
- Being thrown from any motorised and / or moving vehicle.
- Contact sports.
- Diving accidents.
- Falls (greater than patient's own height).
- Head injuries.

Along with the actual cause of injury (history), certain signals suggest head or spinal injury. They include:

SIGNS AND SYMPTOMS OF HEAD OR SPINAL INJURY

A change in consciousness – memory loss, disorientation

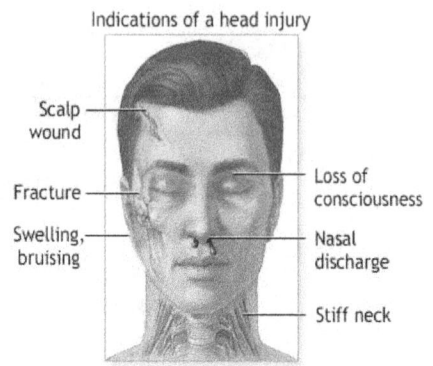

Indications of a head injury

Scalp wound
Fracture
Swelling, bruising
Loss of consciousness
Nasal discharge
Stiff neck

ＡＤＡＭ.

- Pain – headache or point of impact.
- Nausea and / or projectile vomiting.
- Impaired vision.
- Inability to move a body part or weakening of strength.
- Tingling or numbness in hands, fingers, feet and/ or toes.
- Difficult/ depressed breathing.
- Sensory and/ or motor nerve damage.
- The patient often lies on their back with their arms raised above their head (Serious sign).

TREATMENT

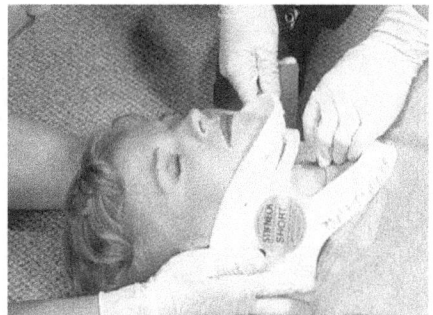

- Stabilise head and neck. Stop movement.
- Maintain an open airway.
- Apply a cervical collar.
- If available, place the casualty on a spinal board (or any improvised surface) by using the log-roll method. Alternatively, activate the EMRS and wait for them to arrive before moving the patient.

It is important to remember that you should never move the patient unless life-threatening factors are present at the location of the emergency.

MANAGING BURNS AND OTHER ENVIRONMENTAL EMERGENCIES

Burn wounds can be extremely painful, and, if not treated correctly, the major concern would be the resulting fluid loss and infection.

As a person is part of the environment that they are in, environmental conditions can have an effect on a person, depending on what the conditions are e.g temperature related conditions (heat or cold), and water related incidences.
In both the above cases, rapid, adequate treatment is vital, in order to prevent the condition of the person from worsening.

CLASSIFICATION OF BURNS

1ST DEGREE / SUPERFICIAL The outer / top layer (epidermis) of skin is affected. Skin is red and dry, swollen and usually painful.	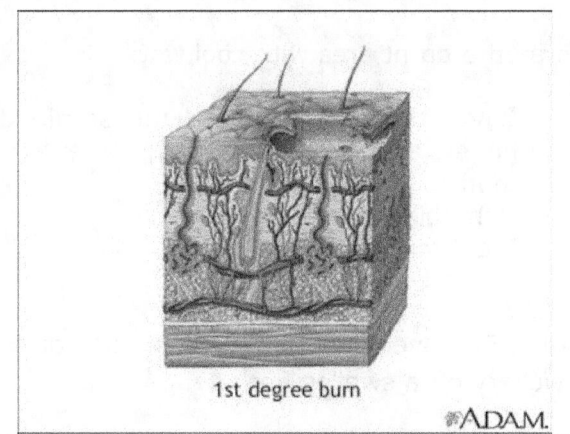 1st degree burn
2ND DEGREE / INTERMEDIATE Top layers are burned. Skin will be red and have blisters. These burns are usually painful.	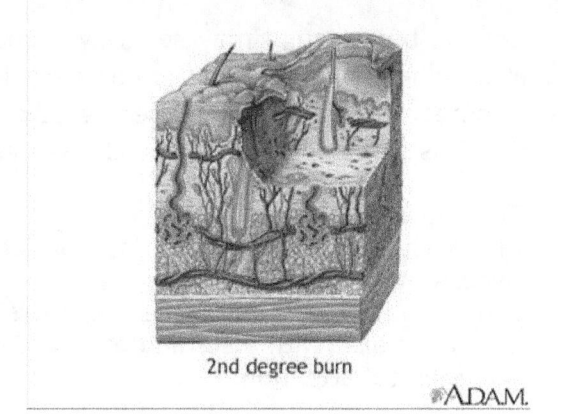 2nd degree burn
3RD DEGREE / DEEP DERMAL All the layers of the skin and underlying tissues (e.g. fat, muscle, bones and nerves) are damaged / destroyed. The skin can appear pale, waxy and / or charred. This type of burn may be quite painful or relatively painless due to nerve destruction.	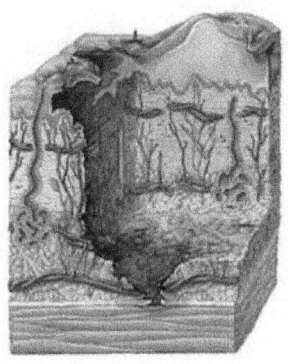 3rd degree burn

TREATMENT

THERMAL BURNS (Flame, Excessive heat, Radiation or sunburns)

Spray the burnt area with cool water

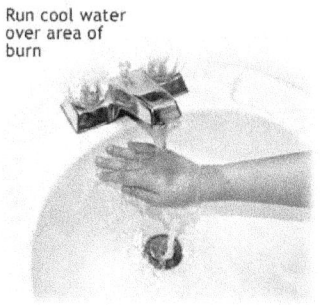

Run cool water over area of burn

- Cover the area with a damp sterile dressing. Should the fingers and toes be involved; place damp dressings between them.
- Immobilise the limb.
- Treat for shock.

Note: Remove rings, jewellery in case of swelling. Do not force jewellery off a swollen finger.

©ADAM.

ELECTRICAL BURNS

An electrical burn wound may severely damage underlying tissue. The patient may have two wounds from an electrical burn (entry / exit site). Never go near a patient who has been electrically burned unless you are sure that it is safe and that the power has been turned off.

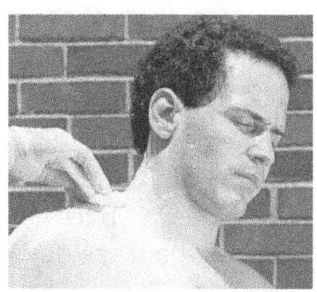

- Turn power source off.
- Check vital signs and provide appropriate cardiac care (if necessary).
- Do not move victim unless necessary (spinal trauma).
- Cover the area with a sterile dressing.
- See medical attention.

CHEMICAL BURNS

There are many chemicals that can cause a burn if they come into contact with skin or mucous membranes. (Example: chlorine, battery acid, DEET, etc.) Chemical burns require immediate care!

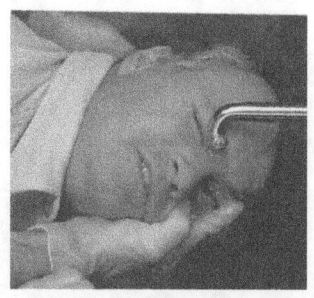

- Wash away the chemical with flowing water (gentle flow of water for at least 20 mins). Avoid hard flushing water pressure.
- Remove contaminated clothing and / or jewellery during flushing procedure.
- If a dry chemical, such as lime, brush away chemical.
- Watch the victim for delayed reactions.
- Chemical in one eye - rinse contaminated eye downward so fluid flows away from other eye.

SMOKE INHALATION

Smoke may irritate or damage the airway. Smoke can cause irritation to the eyes. First priority is to:

- Move patient to a safe area.
- Check vital signs.
- Place victim in a semi-seated or reclined position.
- Call EMRS or call advanced medical help for supplementary oxygen.

Don't for burns care:

- Don't apply any home remedy or ointments.
- Don't apply ice directly on the skin.
- Don't break blisters.
- Don't remove pieces of clothing or any other item stuck to or in the burn.
- Don't give anything to eat or drink, unless he is fully conscious.

Do's for burn care:

- Watch for signs and changes in breathing and consciousness.
- Keep victim from getting chilled or overheated.
- Seek medical attention, if appropriate.

HEAT-RELATED EMERGENCIES

Heat illness follows a continuum. In other words, after the onset of a minor heat illness (if left uncared for), major heat illness will result. It is important to recognize and treat the symptoms of heat illness early to prevent a victim from progressing to heat stroke. In all heat emergencies you will first need to cool the victim down.

Heat Cramps	Heat Exhaustion	Heat Stroke
- Severe muscle cramps. - Moist, cool skin. - Heavy sweating.	- Skin - flushed, cold and clammy. - Heavy sweating. - Pulse – weak. - Headache. - Breathing - Rapid and – Shallow. - Nausea. - Stomach cramps. - Weakness, fatigue.	- Skin - Dry, hot and red. - LOC decreased. - Little or no sweating. - Pulse - full, rapid.
⬇	⬇	⬇
- Remove casualty to a cool place. - Give casualty water with salt/ rehydration fluid. - Pull on cramped muscle. - Massage muscle.	- Remove casualty to a cool place. - Elevate legs. - Remove unnecessary clothing. - Apply cool packs. - Give water. - Monitor!	- Remove casualty to a cool place. -Remove unnecessary clothing. - Sprinkle the casualty with continuously flowing water. - Fan the casualty to further cool him/ her down. - **Call EMRS!** (Life-threatening)

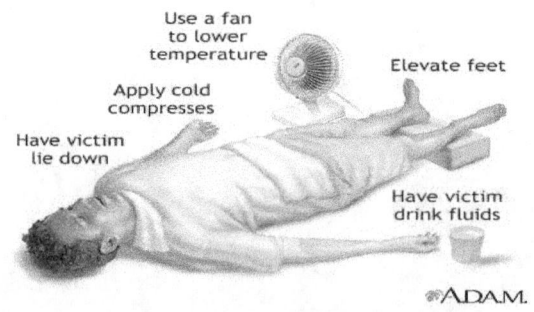

Use a fan to lower temperature

Elevate feet

Apply cold compresses

Have victim lie down

Have victim drink fluids

ADAM.

COLD-RELATED EMERGENCIES

Hypothermia

Hypothermia is the general cooling of the body. It can start off mild and, if uncared for, will develop into severe hypothermia which is life-threatening. The sooner you recognize the signs of hypothermia and provide care, the better the chance is that the condition will not progress. In water the body looses heat 21 times faster than the air at the same ambient temperature. In either case, **SEEK MEDICAL ATTENTION!!** Never give victim alcohol or caffeine to drink!

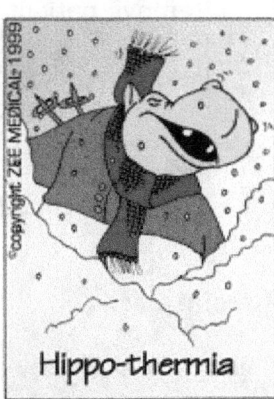

Hippo-thermia

Mild to Moderate Hypothermia

Signs and Symptoms

- Body core temperature 37 °C .... >35 °C.
- Shivering.
- Slurred speech.
- Stumbling or staggering.
- Usually the patient is conscious and can talk.

First Aid Care

- Removal from cold environment.
- Have a source of heat (warm water, fire place).
- Replace wet clothing with dry.
- Provide a hat, blankets, coats, etc. Insulate victim.
- Seek medical attention.

Moderate to Severe Hypothermia

Signs and Symptoms

- Body core temperature <35 °C.
- Shivering has stopped.
- Muscles have become stiff and rigid.
- Skin has a bluish appearance.
- Skin does not react to pain.
- Respiration and pulse slow down.
- Pupils will dilate.
- Victim may appear dead.
- Decreased level of consciousness.
- Failing eye sight.

First Aid Care

- Remove patient from cold environment.
- Remove any wet clothing and replace with dry clothing.
- Passively re-warm the patient (>35°C) - Wrap in a space blanket and give him/her warm drinks (if conscious).
- Have a source of heat (warm water, fire place).
- Provide a hat, blankets, coats, etc. Insulate victim.
- Seek medical attention.

Special Care

Children and elderly patients may be more susceptible to hypothermia and may not show the same signs and symptoms. Children have a low body fat. Older patients may have a higher susceptibility due to loss of fat and decreased efficiency in maintaining normal body temperature.

DROWNING AND NEAR DROWNING

Drowning is defined as death by suffocation under a fluid medium whilst near drowning may be defined as survival following asphyxia or aspiration due to submersion in a fluid medium.

SIGNS AND SYMPTOMS

- WET AND COLD!!
- No responsiveness.
- No Breathing.
- Cyanosis.
- Froth around the casualty's mouth and nostrils.
- Pupils - Dilated and fixed.
- Loss of vital signs.

TREATMENT

- SAFETY! - Throw, tow, row then go, if trained to do so.
- Assess the vital signs.
- CPR, if necessary - CPR is not possible in water. Ventilate the casualty and then move him/ her onto the side of the pool or shore or into a boat. Commence with CPR. With cold water drowning continue with CPR until the EMS arrives.

"A CASUALTY IS NOT DEAD UNTIL WARM AND DEAD"

POISONINGS

A poison is any substance, viz. gas, liquid or solid, that when absorbed, swallowed, inhaled or injected into the body negatively affects the body tissues. Poisonings may be accidental, intentional or forced.

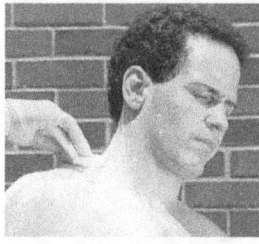 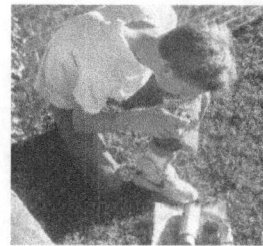 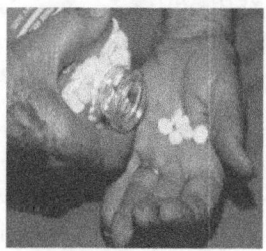 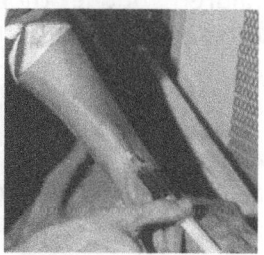

ABSORPTION   **INHALATION**   **INGESTION**   **INJECTION**

SIGNS AND SYMPTOMS

Many of the signs and symptoms of poisonings are the same.

- Difficulty breathing.
- Abdominal pain.
- Headache.
- Nausea and vomiting.
- Neurological dysfunction.
- Excessive salivation and sweating.
- LOC changes (drowsiness ......unconsciousness/ coma).
- Burns, stains and odour in and around the mouth and lips.

TREATMENT

1	Asses the scene for clues and safety. Get patient away from poison, if necessary.
2	Assess victim response (Vital Signs).
3	Provide care for any life-threatening conditions.
4	If patient is conscious, attempt to get more information.
5	Contact Poison Information Centre or local EMRS. Bring any empty container, plant, etc ... to the phone for verification purposes.
6	Follow treatment instructions of Poison Centre.

Do not induce vomiting in the following cases:

- Unconscious or disorientated patients.
- Petroleum/ Paraffin products where ingested.
- Acids/ Alkalis were induced.
- Convulsions.
- Children younger than 1 year old.
- Rattex / similar products ingested.

BITES AND STINGS

There are literally thousands of species of insects capable of stinging. Fortunately, most are not considered to be dangerous. If a stinging victim develops serious symptoms including shortness of breath, flushing, swelling of the face or severe swelling of a body part, further medical attention should be sought immediately. A severe reaction could mean a life-threatening condition is developing - namely, anaphylaxis.

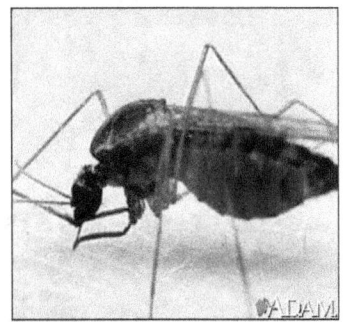

BEE, WASP AND HORNET STINGS

Bees are the only insects that will leave behind a stinger that may remain embedded in the skin. Remove the sting by scraping the sting out with a blade in opposite direction to what the sting is laying. Try not to damage the poison sac. Apply anti-histamine cream and monitor the patient for allergic reaction.

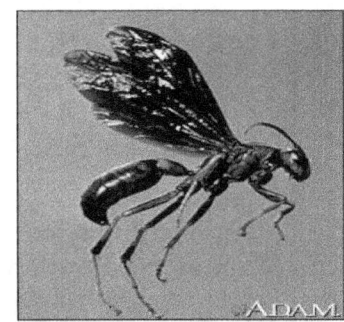

TICKS

Touch the tick with a lit cigarette and it will fall off accordingly. Alternatively you can apply oil over the tick. The oil closes the breathing pores and the tick falls off. Clean the area with soap and water, apply anti-histamine cream. If you are unable to remove the head or if rash persist, obtain medical assistance.

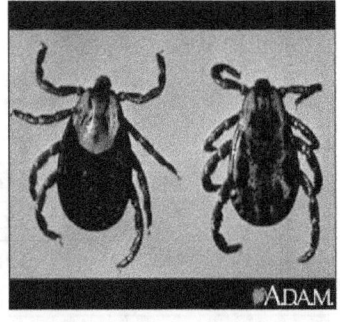

SPIDERS

Try collect/ identify the spider. Disinfect the bite. Apply ice to the bite. Bandage the limb - Distal to proximal. Immobilise the limb.

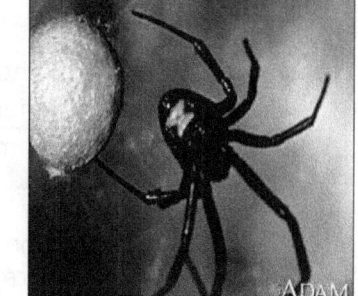

SCORPIONS

Apply ice pack immediately. Disinfect the sting area. Apply ice to the bite. Bandage the limb- Distal to proximal. Immobilise the limb. Monitor the patient for allergic reaction.

SNAKE BITES

SAFETY!! CABC Identify the snake, if possible. Reassure the casualty - keep casualty calm. Bandage the limb, using a firm crepe bandage. Bandage the whole limb, from below the bite wound and towards the heart (distal to proximal). Beware with puff-adder bites due to severe tissue damage and swelling. Should snake venom land in the eyes, rinse thoroughly with a non-irritating liquid (e.g. water). Immobilise the casualty (i.e. patient must not move).

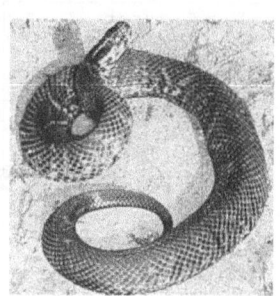

Organizing Assistance

To Organise Emergency Assistance

Emergency Assistance	Call Emergency Services if: • Victim has lost consciousness, is unusually confused, or is losing consciousness; • Victim has difficulty breathing or is not breathing in a normal way; • Has chest pain or pressure that will not go away; • Has persistent pressure or pain in the abdomen; • Is vomiting or is passing blood; • Has seizures, a severe headache, or slurred speech; • Seems to have been poisoned; • Have injuries to his/her head, neck, or back.
Colleagues / Customers	If you ever need to give First Aid, make sure that you get someone to help you. You will need them to call Emergency Services, obtain blankets, or simply stay with the patient while you take any necessary action. Do whatever you have to do to get the attention of someone who can help you – shout, scream, bang on doors or walls. But remember to stay calm and stay in control of the situation.

Back Up Services

Back up services	In the event of an emergency one cannot waste time, so promptly and immediate request assistance and appropriate back up services.
When to Call for Back-up	If someone is injured on Duty the First Aid representative for that area of work should immediately be alerted as well as the HOD and Duty Manager who would make the decision to call the appropriate medical services i.e. ambulance. The incident is then reported to the Regional Safety and Loss Control Manager who then has the responsibility of completing all relevant documentation and keeping all records on file. In the event of injury to the guest, the Duty Manager is immediately contacted and after assessment of situation he/she would alert appropriate medical services i.e. doctor, ambulance, SAP, etc.
Procedures	In the table below find various emergency situations and appropriate back up services to contact:

Emergency Situations	Action
Guests	
Suicide attempts	Report immediately to Duty Manager who will then summon the SAP (South African Police Services) and ambulance services.
Injury	Immediately alert First Aid representative and the Duty Manager.
Illness	Immediately report to the Duty Manager.
Staff	
Injury	Alert first aid representative and Duty Manager ensuring all relevant details of situation documented on the IOD form (Injury On Duty Form).
Illness/heart attack	Same as above.

How to Relay Information to Emergency Units

Suggested practice	When emergency services arrives, you will have to give them the following information:
	
	• **History:**
	  • (What happened) events leading to situation.
	• **Vital signs and symptoms:**
	  • The condition in which you found the patient – the not breathing, no pulse, patient cold, in pain.
	  • What you have done – provide first aid to victim.
	  • As soon as you have done this, get out of the way, but be available for information or assistance if necessary.

Emergency Treatment Sequence Checklist

	Checklist	x	√
1.	**Safety:** of your patient and yourself is of first concern. **Check area for hazardous and safety elements.**		
2.	**Breathing:** are airways clear?		
3.	**Pulse:** CPR needed?		
4.	**Symptoms:** Pain, cold, etc.?		
5.	**Bleeding**: stop and cover wounds.		
6.	**Breaks**: attend to fractures and immobilize them.		
7.	**Transport**: get your patient ready for transport to hospital.		
8.	**Observation**: watch patients respiration, pulse, and movements.		

TRANSPORTATION METHODS

After examination and stabilisation, the patient must be transported. When deciding how to move a patient, the following should be considered:

- The nature of the patient's injuries and specific handling of these injuries, e.g.
  - Spinal injuries.
  - Serious fractures.
- The patient's general condition.
- The resources available.
- Where the patient is located.
  - On a cliff ledge.
  - At sea.

WITHOUT EQUIPMENT

Besides using an ambulance or a stretcher, a patient may be moved by one of the following methods.

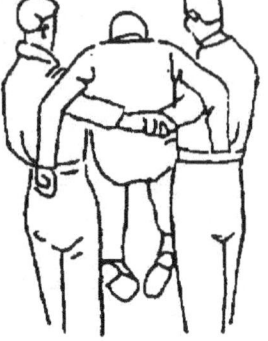

Two-hand seat: Two helpers are needed for this method. The two hand seat can only be used for conscious patients without spinal injuries.

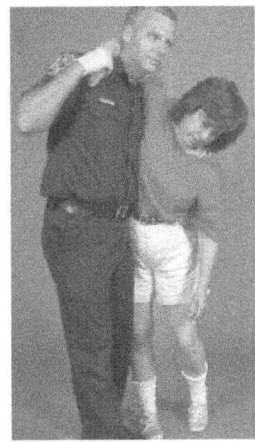

Human crutch: This method is used when the patient finds it difficult to walk alone. The patient places his or her arm around the first aiders neck and he or she is supported while they walk.

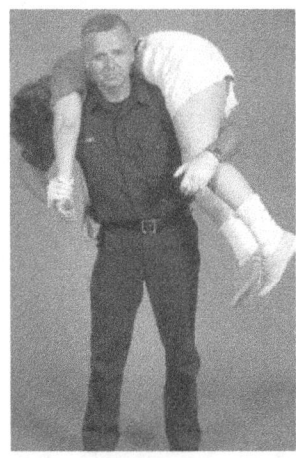

Fireman's Carry: The fireman's carry can only be used for patients without spinal injuries, fractures or dislocations.

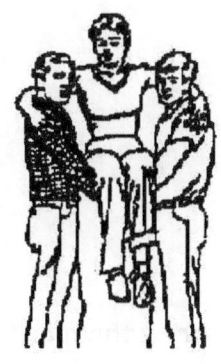

Four-hand seat: Only conscious patients without spinal injuries, fractures or dislocations can be moved using this method. As with the two-hand seat, two helpers are needed.

WITH EQUIPMENT

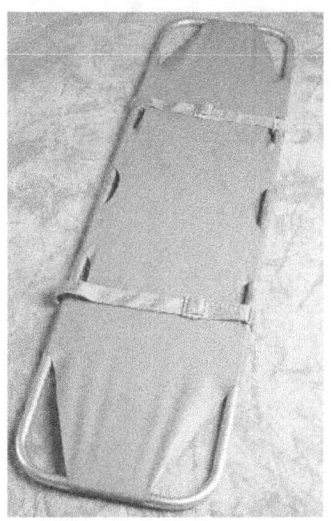

NATO STRETCHER

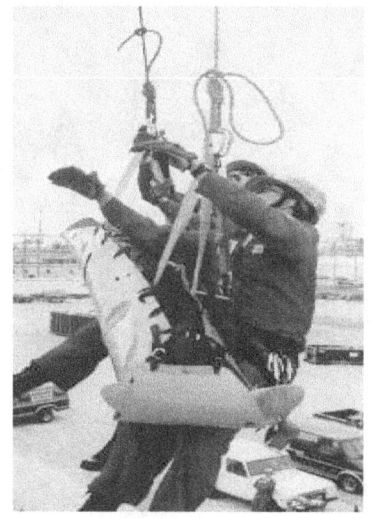

STOKES BASKET

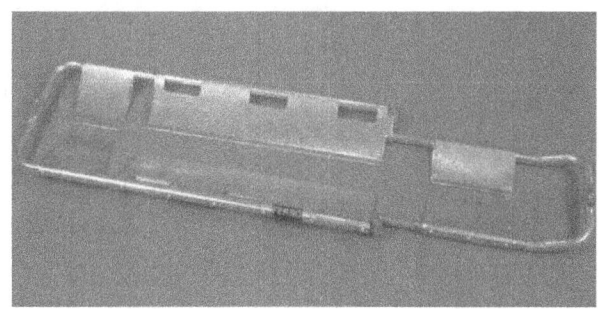

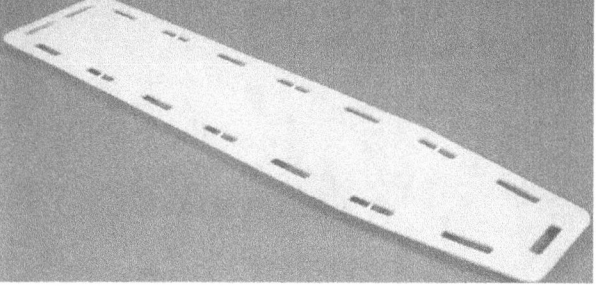

SCOOP STRETCHER   **SPINE BOARD**

IMPROVISED STRETCHERS

- Two poles and a sleeping bag.
- Two poles and two jackets or shirts.
- A blanket rolled up along the sides.

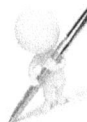

Activity 18: Identify 5 different types of injuries and conditions. Describe them in terms of their severity, cause and possible treatment.

Glossary

Abrasion	A superficial wound in which the topmost layers of the skin are scraped off.
AED	Automated External Defibrillator.
Airway	The passages which transfer air from the outside environment to the lungs; the tracha, bronchi, bronchioles and alveoli.
Artery	A blood vessel carrying blood away from the heart; contains oxygen-rich, high-pressure blood in the systemic cardio-respiratory system.
Avulsion	A tearing away of a section of skin from the layers of tissue beneath it.
Bystander	Any person, trained or untrained, who assists in an emergency situation, but not as part of a duty of employment.
Capillary	The smallest blood vessels in the body; the skin is rife with capillaries.
Carotid artery	The main artery providing blood supply to the head.
Causation	Determination of whether the defendant's actions are causally linked to any harm.
Circulation	The movement of blood throughout the body; performed by the heart.
Consciousness (level of)	A state of awareness or lack thereof.
Consent	A legal condition whereby a person can be said to have given consent based upon an appreciation and understanding of the facts and implications of an action.
CPR	Cardiopulmonary resuscitation.
Cyanosis	The bluish coloration of the skin due to the presence of deoxygenated blood near the skin surface; occurs when the oxygen saturation of arterial blood falls below 85%.
Defibrillation	Delivering a therapeutic dose of electrical energy to the affected heart with a device called a defibrillator.
Diabetes	a disease causing an inability to regulate the level of sugar (glucose) in the blood.
Distal	The point on a limb furthest from its point of attachment to the body.
Duty of Care	A legal obligation imposed on an individual requiring that they exercise a reasonable standard of care while performing any acts that could foreseeable harm others.
EMS	Emergency Medical System.
Hypoxia	A condition in which insufficient oxygen reaches body tissue.

Incision	A clean cut caused by a sharp-edged object.
Insulin	a hormone that allows glucose to travel from the bloodstream into the cells.
Laceration	Irregular wounds caused by a blunt impact to soft tissue which lies over hard tissue; tearing of skin.
Myocardial Infarction	Heart attack; bleeding or blockage cuts off blood flow to part of the heart muscle.
Nail bed	The tissue under the nail; pinching the nail and observing the blood return to the nail bed is a good test of circulation at that location.
Oedema (Edema)	Swelling in the lower legs and ankles. Oedema is caused by a fluid build-up in the body.
Semi-prone position	A position which keeps the tongue from obstructing the airway and allows any fluids to drain from the mouth *(aka recovery position)*.
Standard of Care	The degree of prudence and caution required of an individual who is under a duty of care; the requirements of the standard are closely dependent on circumstances.
Proximal	The point on a limb closest to its point of attachment to the body.
Puncture	A wound caused by an object puncturing the skin.
Vein	A blood vessel that carries blood toward the heart; most veins carry low-oxygen blood.

References

Internet References

http://www.webmd.com/hiv-aids/staying-healthy-10/hiv-aids-treatment

http://en.wikipedia.org/wiki/Management_of_HIV/AIDS

http://www.foundcare.org/HIV-Antiretroviral-Treatment

http://www.fda.gov/ForConsumers/byAudience/ForPatientAdvocates/HIVandAIDSActivities/ucm118915.htm

http://www.scidev.net/sub-saharan-africa/health/hivaids/?gclid=CPr61_X8ob4CFZShtAodnRgA6w

http://www.aidsportal.org/web/guest/home?gclid=CIbn_P_8ob4CFZShtAodnRgA6w

http://www.who.int/occupational_health/5_keys_EN_web.pdf

http://www.who.int/hiv/pub/guidelines/adolescents/en/

www.ingramcontent.com/pod-product-compliance
Lightning Source LLC
Chambersburg PA
CBHW080247180526
45167CB00006B/2446